201
Organic
Smoothies
& Juices

for a

Healthy Pregnancy

Nutrient-Rich Recipes for Your Pregnancy Diet

Nicole Cormier, RD, LDN

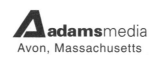
Adamsmedia
Avon, Massachusetts

Published by

Adams Media, a division of F+W Media, Inc.

57 Littlefield Street, Avon, MA 02322. U.S.A.

www.adamsmedia.com

Contains material adapted and abridged from *The Everything® Green Smoothies Book* by Britt Brandon with Lorena Novak Bull, RD, copyright © 2011 by F+W Media, Inc., ISBN 10: 1-4405-2564-1, ISBN 13: 978-1-4405-2564-3; *The Everything® Juicing Book* by Carole Jacobs and Chef Patrice Johnson, technical review by Nicole Cormier, RD, copyright © 2010 by F+W Media, Inc., ISBN 10: 1-4405-0326-5, ISBN 13: 978-1-4405-0326-9; and *The Everything® Pregnancy Nutrition Book* by Kimberly A. Tessmer, RD, LD, copyright © 2005 by F+W Media, Inc., ISBN 10: 1-59337-151-9, ISBN 13: 978-1-59337-151-7.

ISBN 10: 1-4405-5999-6
ISBN 13: 978-1-4405-5999-0
eISBN 10: 1-4405-6000-5
eISBN 13: 978-1-4405-6000-2

Printed in the United States of America.

10   9   8   7   6   5   4   3   2   1

Always follow safety and common-sense cooking protocol while using kitchen utensils, operating ovens and stoves, and handling uncooked food. If children are assisting in the preparation of any recipe, they should always be supervised by an adult.

This book is intended as general information only, and should not be used to diagnose or treat any health condition. In light of the complex, individual, and specific nature of health problems, this book is not intended to replace professional medical advice. The ideas, procedures, and suggestions in this book are intended to supplement, not replace, the advice of a trained medical professional. Consult your physician before adopting any of the suggestions in this book, as well as about any condition that may require diagnosis or medical attention. The author and publisher disclaim any liability arising directly or indirectly from the use of this book.

Many of the designations used by manufacturers and sellers to distinguish their product are claimed as trademarks. Where those designations appear in this book and F+W Media was aware of a trademark claim, the designations have been printed with initial capital letters.

Interior illustration © 123RF.com/Nadiya Struk.

Color photographs © 123RF.com/Inga Nielsen/vanillaechoes/hubavasi/Maksim Shebeko/ildipapp and ©iStockphoto.com/Silberkorn/ivanmateev/cepod

This book is available at quantity discounts for bulk purchases.
For information, please call 1-800-289-0963.

Dedication

This book is dedicated to all moms and moms-to-be.

Acknowledgments

I would like to acknowledge all of the farmers and locavores I have connected with over this past year. You have helped me and the community understand more about where our food comes from and the importance of staying connected to it.

Contents

Introduction   8

Part 1: Pregnancy Smoothies and Juices 101 11
CHAPTER 1: A Healthy Pregnancy Diet. 12
CHAPTER 2: Smoothie and Juicing Essentials 20

Part 2: The Recipes 25
CHAPTER 3: Smoothies 31

Go Bananas. 32
Carrot Top of the Morning to You 33
Apple Pie Smoothie 34
A Berry Great Morning. 35
Mango Tango 36
Orange You Glad You Got Up for This? 37
Splendid Citrus 38
Coconut Craziness. 39
Strawberry Start 40
Luscious Lemon-Lime 41
The Green Go-Getter 42
Pear Splendor 43
A Sweet Beet Smoothie 44
Pleasantly Pear 45
Ginger and Spice Make Everything Nice 46
Mango Madness 47
Calming Cucumber 48

Splendid Melon 49
Tempting Tomato. 50
Super Celery 51
Very Veggie. 52
Go, Go, Garlic!. 53
One Superb Herb. 54
Fresh Start 55
Circulatory Smoothie 56
Stomach Soother. 57
Good Morning Smoothie. 58
Creamy, Nutty, Sweet Smoothie 59
Peas for a Perfect Pregnancy 60
Berry Happy Mama 61
Crazy Carrot 62
Sublime Lime 63
The Pregnancy Helper 64
A Bitter-Sweet Treat. 65

Green Gazpacho 66

Oh, Sweet Cabbage 67

Savoy Smoothie 68

The Slump Bumper 69

Beet Booster 70

Berry, Berry Delicious 71

Peachy Berry 72

Apple-Ginger Delight 73

A Sweet Beet Treat 74

Cool Cucumber Melon 75

A Berry Delicious End to the Day 76

Wacky Watermelon 77

Chocolatey Dream 78

The Joy of Almonds 79

Pumpkin Spice 80

Sweet Potato Pie 81

Coconut Cream Smoothie 82

Sinful Strawberry Cream 83

Raspberry Delight 84

Banana Nut Blend 85

Blueberry Supreme 86

Berry Bananas 87

Go Nuts for Chocolate! 88

Mango Supreme 89

Just Peachy 90

A Daring Pearing 91

Great Granny Smith 92

Veggie Variety 93

A Spicy Assortment 94

Awesome Asparagus 95

Blazing Broccoli 96

Kale Carrot Combo 97

Fantastic Fennel 98

Zippy Zucchini 99

Sweet and Savory Beet 100

The Green Bloody Mary 101

Cabbage Carrot 102

Powerful Pepper Trio 103

Great Garlic 104

Savory Celery Celebration 105

Savory Squash Surprise 106

Turnip Temptation 107

Vitamin C Smoothie 108

Imperative Iron 109

Ginger Melon Stress Meltaway 110

Cabbage, Broccoli, and Celery 111

Raspberry Immune System Smoothie 112

Moodiness Manipulator 113

Pleasurable Pregnancy Smoothie 114

Savory Spinach 115

Maternity Medley 116

Cran-Energy Smoothie 117

Baby, Be Happy 118

Folate-Filled Fruit Smoothie 119

Veggies for Vitamins 120

Refreshing Raspberry Blend 121

Pregnant Pomegranate Smoothie 122

Beta-Carotene Cantaloupe Smoothie 123

Blackberry Delight 124
Romaine Pineapple Smoothie 125
Berry and Banana Smoothie 126
A Grape Way to Bone Health 127
Vitamin C Pack 128

A Cool Blend for Pregnancy 129
Cherry Vanilla Treat 130
Watermelon and Watercress Smoothie 131
Apple Celery Smoothie 132

CHAPTER 4: Juices 133

Kale Apple 134
Carrot Banana 135
Popeye's Rescue 136
Mango Kiwifruit 137
Pineapple Greets Papaya 138
Cabbage Juice 139
Cranberry Apple 140
Watermelon Straight Up 141
Immune Booster 142
Sinus Cleanser 143
Cranberry Orange 144
Strawberry Papaya 145
White Grape and Lime 146
Tropical Cucumber 147
Apple Grape 148
Apple Lemonade 149
Apple Celery 150
Apple Banana 151
Berry Cherry 152
Kale Apple Spinach 153
Ginger Carrot Beet 154
Sunshine in a Glass 155

Cherry Cucumber 156
Papaya Delight 157
Peach Strawberry 158
Dilly of a Cucumber 159
Carrot Apple Broccoli 160
Cherry and Blueberry 161
Lettuce Patch 162
Savoy and Broccoli 163
Carrot Kale 164
Snap Pea Smoothie 165
Salad in a Glass 166
Pineapple Plum Punch 167
Strawberry Patch 168
Purple Cow 169
Strawberry Pineapple Grape 170
Cantaloupe Straight Up 171
Watermelon Lime Cherry 172
Nightcap Smoothie 173
Go to Sleep Smoothie 174
Carrot and Cauliflower 175
Ultimate "C" Energizer 176
Wake Up Watercress Smoothie 177

Orange Lemonade Lift-Off 178

Apple Banana High 179

Razzle Dazzle Berry 180

Pineapple Tangerine 181

Pineapple Cucumber 182

Cauliflower Broccoli 183

Grapefruit Star 184

Broccoli and Kale 185

Spinach Apple 186

Butternut Delight 187

Citrus Cucumber 188

Italian Carrot 189

Ginger Carrot Apple 190

Rise and Shine 191

Apricot Apple 192

Pear Apple 193

Apple Cucumber with a Twist 194

Pear Pineapple 195

Vegetable Seven 196

Broccoli Apple Carrot 197

Garlic Delight 198

Carrot, Cucumber, and Beet 199

Super Berry 200

Carrots in the Veggie Patch 201

Apple Blackberry 202

A Pear of Kiwifruit 203

Peach Grape Delight 204

Fresh from the Garden 205

Tangy Cucumber 206

Orange Broccoli 207

String Bean Juice 208

Carrot Cauliflower 209

Broccoli Carrot 210

Apple Cabbage 211

Cucumber Melon Pear 212

Green Apple Broccoli 213

Peach Pineapple 214

Apple Grapefruit 215

Cucumber Pepper 216

Asparagus Squash Medley 217

Super Green Juice 218

Kiwifruit Apple 219

Orange Carrot 220

Berry Melon 221

Cucumber Lemonade 222

Super Melon 223

Blueberry Banana 224

Apple Beeter 225

Celery Carrot 226

Watermelon Orange 227

Broccoli Cabbage Patch 228

Green Juice 229

Carrot Beeter 230

Piece of Pie 231

Apple Yammer 232

Garlic Melon with Sprig of Dill 233

Index   234

Introduction

How can smoothies and juices help you sail through the nine months of pregnancy stress-free? Well, maybe you suffer from low energy or morning sickness? Maybe you're concerned that you're not eating the right foods to make sure your baby-to-be develops healthy bones or a strong nervous system? Maybe those pregnancy cravings have you up in the middle of the night scrounging through your fridge looking for something (anything!) that will hit the spot?

Fortunately, the 201 recipes for organic smoothies and juices found throughout this book will help you calm those cravings, quell that morning sickness, and feel good knowing that you're giving your baby all the vitamins, minerals, and nutrients he needs to grow healthy and strong.

In Part 1 you'll learn everything you need to know about why you should choose organic, how juices and smoothies can help you—and your baby!—get all the nutrients you need during your pregnancy, and what you need to create all the smoothies and juices found throughout the book.

In Part 2 you'll find recipes for 201 organic, nutrient-filled smoothies and juices and information about how these recipes can be particularly beneficial over the next nine months. The recipes' ingredients run the gamut from sweet to savory and each will do something different for your body and your baby, such as the Turnip Temptation that will help your baby's developing nervous system, the Blackberry Delight that will strengthen both you and your baby's immune systems, and the Pumpkin Spice that will help keep your digestive system on track.

So get your blenders ready and your juicers powered up! You only have nine short months to enjoy all the benefits these smoothies and juices have to offer and you don't want to miss a single sip. Enjoy!

PART 1

Pregnancy Smoothies and Juices 101

So why should you go organic during your pregnancy? What nutrients do you really need to take in on a regular basis, and how much more of each do you need while you're pregnant? How do you make smoothies and juices, anyway? This Part answers all those questions and more to help you know what you need for the healthiest pregnancy possible—for both you *and* your baby-to-be.

CHAPTER 1
A Healthy Pregnancy Diet

A healthy pregnancy diet needs a balance of dietary components that pack as many nutrients per calorie as possible. These nutrient-dense calories are key to a healthy pregnancy. One way to increase your intake of nutrient-dense calories during pregnancy is to add the right kind of juices and smoothies into your diet. These tasty additions pack in important macro- and micronutrients essential to a healthy pregnancy.

As your baby is growing, so will your caloric needs. On average, the caloric needs of a pregnant woman will increase by around 300 calories a day. In order to make sure you are getting the most of each of those calories, you want to make sure they are packed with the necessary nutrients for a healthy pregnancy, such as folic acid, calcium, and iron.

There are a number of different benefits and sources for these pregnancy nutrients. Here's a brief overview as to why these nutrients are important during pregnancy and what types of foods provide them.

Folic Acid

Folate, found naturally in foods, is one of the B vitamins; it is also known as folic acid. During pregnancy, this vitamin helps to properly develop the neural tube, which becomes the baby's spine. When taken in daily optimal amounts at least one month before becoming pregnant and during the first trimester, folic acid can help prevent birth defects of the brain and spinal cord, called neural tube defects (NTDs). Though the Institute of Medicine of the National Academies still states that the recommended intake is 400 micrograms (mcg) for women of childbearing age, recent studies show that to decrease the risk of birth defects, folic acid should be increased to 800–1000 mcg daily (the amount in most prenatal vitamins) in those who are pregnant or are attempting to become pregnant. So your doctor will likely prescribe a prenatal vitamin with this higher amount.

Because most women do not know that they are pregnant right away and because the neural tube and the brain begin to form so quickly after conception, taking optimal amounts of folic acid on a daily basis is important for all women in their childbearing years.

GOOD SOURCES OF FOLIC ACID

- **Cranberries.** High in vitamins C, B complex, and A, and folic acid, cranberries help prevent bladder infections by keeping bacteria from clinging to the wall of the bladder.

- **Pears.** Rich in fiber, vitamins B and C, folic acid, niacin, and the minerals phosphorus and calcium, pears help your bladder and constipation.

- **Oranges.** A rich source of vitamins C, B, and K; biotin; folic acid; amino acids; and minerals, oranges cleanse the gastrointestinal tract, strengthen capillary walls, and benefit the heart and lungs.

- **Apples.** Rich in vitamins A, B_1, B_2, B_6, and C; folic acid; biotin; and a host of minerals that promote healthy skin, hair, and nails, apples also contain pectin, a fiber that absorbs toxins, stimulates digestion, and helps reduce cholesterol.

Other B Vitamins

Vitamin B_6 is necessary in helping your body make nonessential amino acids (the building blocks of protein). These nonessential amino acids are used to make necessary body cells. Vitamin B_6 also helps to turn the amino acid tryptophan into niacin and serotonin (a messenger in the brain). In addition to those functions, this vitamin helps produce insulin, hemoglobin, and antibodies that help fight infection. Requirements are increased slightly in pregnancy due to the needs of the baby. The recommended level during pregnancy is 1.9 milligrams (mg).

Requirements are also increased for vitamin B_{12} during pregnancy to help with the formation of red blood cells. The increase is slight, from 2.4mcg before pregnancy to 2.6mcg during pregnancy.

Calcium

Calcium is a mineral that deserves special attention throughout a woman's life, especially when it comes to pregnancy. Calcium is important for strong bones and teeth, a healthy heart, nerves, muscles, and the development of normal heart rhythm and blood-clotting abilities. Not consuming enough calcium and/or not having good calcium stores will force the baby to use calcium from your own bones. Consuming plenty of calcium before, during, and after pregnancy can also help to reduce your risk for osteoporosis, or brittle bone disease, later in life.

Intake Requirements

Whether pregnant or not, calcium needs for teens (age fourteen to eighteen) is 1,300mg and 1,000mg for woman age nineteen to fifty. Women older than fifty need 1,200mg of calcium daily. The tolerable upper intake level for calcium is 2,500mg daily.

GOOD SOURCES OF CALCIUM

- **Grapefruit.** Rich in vitamin C, calcium, phosphorus, and potassium as well, grapefruit helps strengthen capillary walls and reduce indigestion, varicose veins, obesity, and morning sickness.

- **Strawberries.** Strawberries are packed with vitamin C, iron, calcium, magnesium, folate, and potassium—essential for immune system function and for strong connective tissue.

- **Broccoli.** Packed with fiber to help regularity, broccoli is also surprisingly high in protein, and it's full of calcium, antioxidants, and vitamins B$_6$, C, and E.

- **Beets.** Both the beet greens and beet roots are juiceable and highly nutritious. The roots are packed with calcium, potassium, and vitamins A and C.

Iron

Iron is another essential mineral that merits special attention as part of your diet before and during pregnancy. Iron is essential to the formation of healthy red blood cells, which are responsible for carrying oxygen through your blood to the cells of your body. Almost two-thirds of the iron in your body is found in hemoglobin, the protein in red blood cells that carries oxygen to your body's tissues. The increase in blood volume that takes place during pregnancy greatly increases a woman's need for iron. If you do not get enough iron and/or do not have adequate iron stores, the growing baby will take it at your expense. Iron deficiency during pregnancy can cause anemia, extreme fatigue, a low birth-weight baby, and other potential problems.

The greater your iron stores before you become pregnant, the better iron will be absorbed during pregnancy.

Intake Requirements

During pregnancy, your iron requirement climbs from 18mg for women between nineteen and fifty years old to 27mg per day. Again, as with many other vitamins and minerals, too much iron is not always best. Iron has a tolerable upper intake level of 45mg. Foods that supply iron include meat, poultry, fish, legumes, and whole-grain and enriched grain products. Iron from plant sources (or "nonheme iron") is not as easily absorbed as that from animal sources (or "heme iron"). Supplementing your meals with a beverage rich in vitamin C, such as citrus fruits or juices, broccoli, tomatoes, or kiwi, will help your body better absorb the iron in the foods you consume.

GOOD SOURCES OF IRON

- **Radishes.** Small but mighty in taste and loaded with vitamin C, iron, magnesium, and potassium, radish juice cleanses the nasal sinuses and gastrointestinal tract and helps clear up skin disorders.

- **Spinach, kale, and Swiss chard.** Popeye was right all along. You'll be strong to the finish if you eat your spinach, kale, and chard, which are similar in nutritional value and provide ample supplies of iron, phosphorus, fiber, and vitamins A, B, C, E, and K.

- **Lettuce.** Deep-green lettuce is a good source of calcium, chlorophyll, iron, magnesium, potassium silicon, and vitamins A and E. All types help rebuild hemoglobin, add shine and thickness to hair, and promote hair growth.

Beta-Carotene

Vitamin A promotes the growth and health of cells and tissues for both the mother and the baby and, in the form of beta-carotene, vitamin A also acts as a powerful antioxidant. Beta-carotene, which forms vitamin A, does not pose any danger to expectant mothers. However, too high of doses of the preformed vitamin A, not beta-carotene, can cause birth defects and liver toxicity.

Your body easily converts beta-carotene to vitamin A only when the body needs it. The recommended daily allowance (RDA) of vitamin A is measured in micrograms (mcg). In supplements and on nutrition facts panels, it is measured in international units (IU). The need for vitamin A increases only slightly during pregnancy, from 700 to 770mcg (for women nineteen to fifty years of age), which adds up to 2,334 to 2,567 IU.

GOOD SOURCES OF BETA-CAROTENE

- Carrots
- Mangos
- Spinach
- Squash

Vitamin D

Another important fat-soluble vitamin that's essential during pregnancy is vitamin D. This vitamin aids in calcium balance and helps your body absorb sufficient calcium for you and your baby. Vitamin D is known as the sunshine vitamin because the body can make vitamin D after sunlight hits the skin. It is important to get enough vitamin D throughout your life as a way of helping to avoid osteoporosis (or brittle bone disease). Since vitamin D is stored in the body, too much can be toxic. Toxic levels of vitamin D usually come from supplements, not food sources or sunlight. During pregnancy, women should get 5mcg or 200 IU per day.

GOOD SOURCES OF VITAMIN D

- Sunflower seeds
- Sprouts
- Mushrooms
- Fortified milk, including cows' milk, almond, soy, and rice

Vitamin C

Vitamin C produces collagen, a connective tissue that holds muscles, bones, and other tissues together. In addition it helps with a variety of other functions, including forming and repairing red blood cells, bones, and other tissue; protecting you from bruising; and boosting your immune system.

> ## GOOD SOURCES OF VITAMIN C
>
> - **Watermelon.** It is very high in electrolytes and vitamin C. It will help re-energize you, especially if you're working out during your pregnancy.

Zinc

Almost every cell in the body contains zinc, which is also part of over seventy different types of enzymes. Zinc is known as the second most abundant trace mineral in the human body. Your requirement for this mineral increases slightly during pregnancy from 8 to 11 mg (for women nineteen to fifty years). Zinc is needed for cell growth and brain development. Too much iron from supplements can inhibit the absorption of zinc.

Women who are having multiple babies have slightly higher recommended intakes for some vitamins and minerals. Your doctor can advise you as to your recommended nutritional intake.

> ## GOOD SOURCES OF ZINC
>
> - **Broccoli.** It is rich in vitamins A, B, C, and K; fiber; zinc; folic acid; magnesium; iron; and beta-carotene.

Sodium

Although sodium sometimes gets bad press, it is still a mineral that is essential to life and to good health—and that also means during pregnancy.

Sodium has many important functions in the body, such as controlling the flow of fluids in and out of each cell, regulating blood pressure, transmitting nerve impulses, and helping your muscles relax (including the heart, which is a muscle). Sodium chloride and potassium are known as electrolytes, compounds that transmit electrical currents through the body. As a result of these currents, nerve impulses can also be transmitted.

Recommended Amounts

The terms "salt" and "sodium" are often used interchangeably, yet they are two different things. Sodium is an element of table salt, which is technically known as sodium chloride. How much sodium is in table salt? A single teaspoon of salt contains 2,000mg of sodium. Generally, articles and guidelines that warn of the dangers of eating too much salt are concerned with sodium only.

YOUR PREGNANCY DIET

A healthy diet will ensure that you and your baby receive the necessary nutrients that are essential for you both during pregnancy. This overview of important prenatal vitamins and minerals is a great first step to remaining healthy during pregnancy. In addition, you should consult with your doctor about dietary guidelines for your pregnancy. You can then work these delicious and nutritious smoothies and juices into your diet as you see fit.

CHAPTER 2

Smoothie and Juicing Essentials

When it comes to making your own smoothies and juices, there are a few things you need to remember about both tasty beverages. Proper preparation and selection of both ingredients and equipment is key. As a standard for these recipes, choosing organic ingredients is preferable, as they are a healthier alternative to conventionally grown fruits and vegetables. There is more information on the benefits of organic produce later in the chapter—but first, let's go over some important decisions and instructions for making your own smoothies and juicing on your own.

MAKING YOUR OWN SMOOTHIES

In order to prepare a smoothie, all that's needed are the fruits and vegetables of your choosing (according to recipes that sound appetizing to you) and a high-speed blender capable of emulsifying the ingredients.

Choosing the Right Blender

The blender needed for smoothies can be completely based on your needs and choosing. In most reviews of blenders on the market today, smoothie consumers compare them based upon a few major factors: power, noise, capacity, and ease of cleanup.

- **Power.** The power of your blender will determine how quickly and efficiently your smoothie and its ingredients can be liquefied and blended. If time or texture are of no importance, this factor may not require much attention.
- **Noise.** Noise can be of no importance or of the utmost importance when it comes to selecting the perfect blender. If you plan on blending your smoothie prior to the rest of your house waking, it might be smart to invest in a quieter version that will still get the job done nicely.
- **Capacity.** Capacity is extremely important, considering you will be putting cups of fruits and vegetables, along with other ingredients, into the same canister. You will need enough room for the blending to be efficient. Also, be sure to take into consideration that you will need enough room in your blender for the adequate amount of ingredients for your desired number of servings.
- **Ease of cleanup.** Although cleanup may also seem like a nonissue at first thought, consider your schedule or routine when making this purchase. Do you need it to be dishwasher-safe? Will the blender require special tools for cleaning? Is there a recommended strategy to keep the blender clean while also ensuring a long lifespan?

Whether you'd like to use your tried-and-true kitchen blender or you'd rather opt for a high-horsepower emulsifying machine, the choice is yours.

Selecting and Storing Your Ingredients and Smoothies

The prep time required for the ingredients starts as soon as you get your greens, fruits, and vegetables home. Although greens will remain green for days or weeks, their powerful antioxidants, vitamins, and minerals dissipate from the time of picking, so eating them as soon as possible ensures you are getting the most nutrition out of every ounce.

A cutting board, peeler, and knife will help in cleaning and preparing your fruits and vegetables with ease and assist in quick cleanup. In most cases, you will want to soak and rinse your ingredients in cold water, but rinsing by hand can be done just as easily. Lettuces and greens should be washed and stored in an airtight bag or container with paper towels or something that can dry excess water off the leaves. Some vegetables such as carrots, turnips, and beets should be rid of their stems and green tops in order to prevent drying the vegetables out. Both fruits and vegetables with hard outer skins or rinds should be peeled prior to blending, and pits should always be removed.

After blending your smoothie, you can take it on the go in any insulated container that will help maintain its temperature and freshness, or you can store it in an airtight glass container in your refrigerator for up to three days.

The simplicity of smoothies is found in what is required to create one: a blender, a knife for food prep, and the fruits and vegetables of your choosing. That's it!

JUICING ON YOUR OWN

Nothing quite hits the spot like a freshly made glass of juice—whether you're pregnant or not. Fruits and vegetables provide a wealth of nutritional benefits that could never be squeezed into a vitamin supplement. Also, no other health food on earth can be so quickly digested and absorbed by the body.

Gearing Up for Juicing

Juicing is extremely simple, but it pays to invest in a quality juicer and learn the ins and outs of juicing techniques before attempting to create your own beverages.

Like any home appliance, your juicer will last much longer if you respect its size, limitations, and quirks, and keep it clean and in good working order after each use. If you're buying a used model, you may want to have a veteran juicer look it over before you use it for the first time. The last thing you want to do is butcher fruits and vegetables and render them useless for your juices. Plus, it's always better to be safe than sorry when it comes to dealing with appliances that have motors and sharp blades.

Juicing Dos and Don'ts

Here are a few tips and trade secrets to ensure smooth juicing:

- Wash all produce before juicing. Remove bruises, mold, blemishes, and dings.
- Go organic. The price is more than worth the health benefits. Otherwise, you'll have to peel everything before placing it in the juicer and lose out on lots of nutrients. Non-organic produce is sprayed with pesticides that penetrate the peels and skins of produce—the largest source of nutrients in produce.
- Always peel oranges, tangerines, bananas, avocados, kiwifruits, pineapples, and grapefruit, even if they're organic.
- Don't remove the stems and leaves of most produce, including beet stems and leaves, strawberry caps, and small grape stems. They contain a high concentration of nutrients and won't hurt you or your juicer.
- Cut most fruits and vegetables into strips or sections that fit easily into your juicer's tube without forcing or jamming. With experience, you'll learn what size works best for your particular machine.
- Insert a grocery store–sized plastic bag in the pulp receptacle of your juicer to catch the pulp during juicing. When you've finished making your juice, you can either throw away the pulp, or save it for cooking or composting, and there's no need to wash the pulp receptacle after each use.

Since all juicers are a little bit different, be sure to read the instructions carefully and follow them closely. The last thing you would want to do is have an accident.

GO ORGANIC

Whenever possible, use organic fruits and vegetables for your smoothies and juices. Organic produce is grown without synthetic fertilizers and chemical biocides. Every year, the conventional U.S. agriculture industry goes through more than 1 billion pounds of pesticides and herbicides. Only 2 percent of that actually kills insects; the remaining 98 percent goes into the soil, air, water, and food supply—including the nonorganic fruits and veggies you eat! Buying and consuming organic produce is one way to circumvent this health hazard.

Because organic farming does not use chemicals to preserve produce, it focuses on growing crops in season. By using organic produce grown in the United States and close to your home, you'll use fruits and vegetables that are grown in season rather than imported from foreign countries where organic standards may not be as high and where carcinogenic sprays are still legal.

No chemicals or pesticides are used in the organic growing process. In 2002, the National Organic Program, administered by the U.S. Department of Agriculture, prohibited the use of chemicals in organic farming and stipulated management practices "with an intent to restore and then maintain ecological harmony on the farm, its surrounding environment, and ultimately, the whole planetary ecosystem." It's important to know that some small farms cannot afford or don't have enough time to go through the certification process, but do grow organically.

It's especially important to buy organic when purchasing produce that is particularly vulnerable to pesticide contamination. This includes apples, apricots, bell peppers, cherries, celery, grapes, green beans, cucumbers, peaches, spinach, and strawberries.

You should also steer clear of produce that's been irradiated, or subjected to gamma ray radiation to kill pests and germs and prolong shelf life. Irradiation can lead to the formation of dangerous chemicals in produce called radiolytic products, which include formaldehyde and benzene.

Be on the Lookout

When choosing organic produce in the grocery store, look for labels marked "certified organic." This guarantees that the produce has been grown according to the strict standards set forth by the National Organic Program, including inspection of farms and processing facilities, detailed record keeping, and testing the soil and water for pesticides to ensure government standards are met. Labels reading "transitional organic" mean the food was grown on a farm that has recently converted or is in the process of converting from conventional to organic farming practices.

PART 2

The Recipes

Now that you know what to eat and why, it's time to start blending some smoothies and mixing up some nutrient-rich juices. In this Part, you'll find 201 organic, nutrient-packed recipes that will help make the next nine months absolutely delicious! The smoothies and juices that are especially helpful for common pregnancy symptoms, such as morning sickness or a lack of energy, or common pregnancy concerns such as fetal development, are marked with recipe callouts (discussed on the following pages) to help you get the most from each and every sip. Enjoy!

RECIPE CALLOUTS

Throughout this part you'll find callouts for smoothie and juice recipes that are especially good for you throughout your pregnancy. These callouts indicate recipes that offer the following benefits:

Good for your baby's nervous system

Your baby's nervous system begins to develop around week 3 of gestation when the spinal cord begins to form. Folate, or folic acid, one of the B vitamins, is an important nutrient that will support a healthy and functioning nervous system. Folate is found in a variety of foods, including spinach, broccoli, beets, strawberries, and tomatoes. Drinking smoothies and juices with these ingredients will allow you to consume at least 400mcg, the recommended amount during pregnancy.

Good for morning sickness

In the first trimester, three-quarters of pregnant women experience morning sickness, with nausea and/or vomiting. It can happen at any time of day at different intensities, leaving you feeling exhausted and miserable. A combination of many physical changes taking place in your body is the main contributor of morning sickness. These smoothies and juices may contain ginger, which has been shown to bring relief. In addition, watermelon may also help alleviate morning sickness due to its water content and raspberries have been used for centuries to treat morning sickness and may also be present in some of these smoothies or juices.

Good for your digestive system

Your digestion will be affected during pregnancy and the most common symptom is constipation. During pregnancy, food passes more slowly through your intestines due to hormones that cause the muscles of the digestive tract to relax. In addition, your uterus can also press on the colon, causing similar effects. The good news is that fruits and vegetables that contain more fiber have been shown to help constipation, as long as you consume plenty of fluids. Some types of produce—including watercress, beets, cabbage, carrots, tomatoes, and watermelon—are also diuretics, which mean that they contain a high water content that helps flush out toxins. In addition, water-filled cucumbers are rich in sulfur and silicon that help remove uric acid. The fiber content or diuretic impact of the smoothies and juices marked with this callout will help with constipation and help you maintain a healthy digestive system throughout your pregnancy.

Good for pregnancy cravings

A pregnant woman's cravings for pickles and ice cream have been the premise of many a joke and many women do experience unusual cravings during pregnancy. You can avoid overeating during these cravings by making sure you're taking in enough fiber. Making this an important part of your diet is one way to manage blood sugars that will help control your hunger and energy levels: It slows your digestion, therefore your blood sugars will be more balanced. These juices can help you curb your cravings from the abundance of nutrients they provide, and some may even satisfy your cravings.

Helps boost energy levels

The level of stress on your body during pregnancy can lead to exhaustion. There is a reason they say, "You're now eating for two." Your metabolism will increase during pregnancy, urging you to eat more vitamins and minerals for your growing baby. Incorporating the smoothies and juices marked with this callout will help prevent vitamin and mineral deficiencies throughout your pregnancy. These smoothies and juices contain a higher amount of electrolytes, vitamin C, or B vitamins, all of which will give your energy a bump in the right direction. Electrolytes promote hydration, which is known to improve energy levels; vitamin C has a high amount of antioxidants that reduces stress in the body, therefore it increase metabolic rate and maintains energy levels; and B vitamins aid in energy production by assisting with the metabolism of carbohydrates, proteins, and fats. B_6 and B_{12} deficiencies are known to lead to lethargy, so bulk up on melons and leafy greens, which are known to contain these vitamins.

Good for healthy skin and hair

During pregnancy your changing hormones can wreak havoc on your skin. The smoothies and juices marked with this callout are full of vitamins A, C, and E; these vitamins are antioxidants that help repair damaged tissue and support the growth of new cells, and they will improve your skin and put a beautiful shine in your hair.

Good for your baby's bones and development

A healthy diet is essential for the development of your baby. There are a few key nutrients that add extra support to ensure your baby's bones, teeth, red blood cells, and muscles develop adequately—especially during the second trimester. They include vitamins A, E, and C; calcium; and magnesium. Magnesium and calcium work together to support strong bones and vitamin C helps out with bone growth and repair, and the formation of collagen that is the foundation of bone health. These recipes also help decrease the likelihood of birth defects, the majority of which occur during the first trimester. It is recommended to reach 400mg of folic acid daily to reduce the risk of birth defects of the brain and spine. These smoothies and juices will help you meet your daily requirements for the vitamins A, C, and E; calcium; magnesium; and folate.

Good for strengthening your immune system

Your immune system is made up of cells, tissues, and organs that have to be protected to decrease the risk of illnesses. Overall, your immune system's basic task is to protect you and your baby from any foreign free radicals that may cause harm. The stronger your immune system, the more protection you'll have against these. These smoothies and juices contain higher levels of vitamin C which, in combination with vitamins A and E, minerals such as selenium and zinc, and flavonoids, support your immune system and help repair tissues. Vitamin C is an antioxidant that specifically protects tissues from damage. It also helps your body absorb iron, which is required for the production of hemoglobin and prevents anemia.

Good for fighting infections during pregnancy

There are several infections that women are more susceptible to during pregnancy. The most common are urinary tract, bladder, and yeast infections, which occur due to changes in the urinary tract. In addition, the growth of your uterus can block some of your urine from draining, which may lead to an infection. Cranberries are a well-known remedy for infections, because they produce hippuric acid in the urine that prevents bacteria from sticking to the walls of the bladder. Vitamin C, beta-carotene, and zinc can also help fight these infections. These smoothies and juices will support your recovery from these infections.

CHAPTER 3
Smoothies

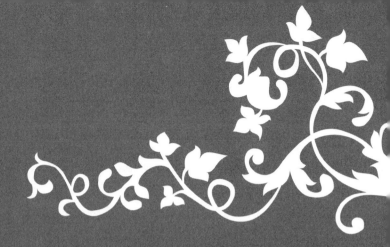

From the Green Go-Getter and the Kale Carrot Combo to the Mango Madness and Cherry Vanilla Treat, this selection of delicious smoothies makes every calorie count. Some are a little more sweet and others a bit more savory, but all offer a tasty way to get those nutrients necessary for a healthy pregnancy.

Go Bananas

Helps boost energy levels

This potassium-rich smoothie will leave you feeling energized by supporting fluid and electrolyte balance in your cells. Since your blood volume expands by up to 50 percent during pregnancy, your electrolyte needs also increase . . . and this smoothie will help keep the extra fluid in the right chemical balance.

YIELDS: 1 QUART

2 cups spinach leaves
2 ripe bananas, peeled
1 apple, peeled and cored
1 cup purified water

1. Combine spinach, bananas, apple, and ½ cup water in a blender and blend thoroughly.
2. While blending, add remaining water until desired texture is achieved.

	Calories	Fat	Protein	Sodium	Fiber	Carbohydrates
PER 1 CUP SERVING	75	0g	1g	14mg	2g	19g

A NATURAL THICKENING AGENT?

Because bananas have such a low water content, they can be used as a great natural alternative to common thickening agents. You can actually watch the bananas take a liquefied smoothie and turn it into a delightfully thickened version. Experiment and watch as the banana thickens the smoothie before your very eyes!

Carrot Top of the Morning to You

Good for your baby's bones and development

Rich in beta-carotene, this smoothie is particularly essential for women who are about to give birth, because it helps to repair postpartum tissue. Vitamins A and C also play key roles in encouraging bone growth. They also help the development of the heart, lungs, kidneys, eyes, and bones, and the circulatory, respiratory, and central nervous systems of your baby-to-be.

YIELDS: 1 QUART

2 cups romaine lettuce, shredded

3 carrots, peeled and cut into sticks suitable for blender's ability

1 apple, peeled and cored

1 cup purified water

1. Combine first 3 ingredients in the order listed in a blender.
2. Add water slowly while blending until desired texture is achieved.

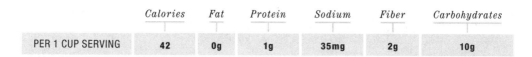

	Calories	Fat	Protein	Sodium	Fiber	Carbohydrates
PER 1 CUP SERVING	42	0g	1g	35mg	2g	10g

Apple Pie Smoothie

Good for pregnancy cravings

The cloves and cinnamon in this smoothie add a flavor reminiscent of apple pie, which can be useful if you're experiencing cravings for sweets or feel like a nighttime treat, and the fiber alone may help your body feel balanced. Healthy *and* delicious? Indeed!

YIELDS: 1 QUART

2 cups spinach

1 teaspoon cloves

1 teaspoon cinnamon

3 apples, peeled and cored

1½ cups coconut milk

1. Layer the spinach in the blender's container.
2. Add the spices, followed by the apples.
3. Add milk slowly while blending until desired texture is achieved.

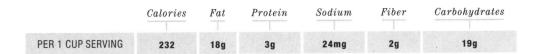

	Calories	Fat	Protein	Sodium	Fiber	Carbohydrates
PER 1 CUP SERVING	232	18g	3g	24mg	2g	19g

THE SURPRISING POWER OF CLOVES

Although most consider cloves an essential when it comes time to make pies for the holidays, Ayurvedic healers utilize this spice for its healing powers—it's believed to alleviate symptoms of irregular digestion and headaches, which can be common during pregnancy. Although cloves are only used in small amounts, their antibacterial and antiviral properties in any amount can't hurt and could keep you from having to take any medications during your pregnancy!

A Berry Great Morning

Helps boost energy levels

This smoothie is packed with rich antioxidants, powerful phytochemicals, and loads of protein that will get you through a busy day of doctor's appointments. Soymilk is safe to drink during pregnancy and some soymilks have omega-3 fatty acids, which are long-chain polyunsaturated fatty acids that reduce inflammation and are essential for health.

YIELDS: 1 QUART

2 cups mixed baby greens

1 pint raspberries

1 pint blueberries

1 banana, peeled

1 cup vanilla soymilk

1. Combine greens, berries, and banana and blend thoroughly.
2. While blending, add soymilk slowly until desired texture is achieved.

	Calories	Fat	Protein	Sodium	Fiber	Carbohydrates
PER 1 CUP SERVING	94	2g	3g	28mg	6g	19g

Smoothies

Mango Tango

Helps boost energy levels

This fruity blend will leave you energized with its combo of vitamins C, A, and B_6 and folic acid. It will help you conquer the most hectic morning!

½ cup dandelion greens

1 cup iceberg lettuce

1 ripe mango, peeled and
   pit removed

1 cup pineapple, cubed

1 orange, peeled

½ cup purified water

1. Combine dandelion greens, iceberg, mango, pineapple, and orange with ¼ cup water and blend thoroughly.
2. While blending, add remaining water until desired texture is achieved.

	Calories	Fat	Protein	Sodium	Fiber	Carbohydrates
PER 1 CUP SERVING	79	0g	1g	9mg	2g	20g

Orange You Glad You Got Up for This?

Good for strengthening your immune system

This vitamin C booster can help prevent vitamin C deficiencies in your baby, which has been related to impairing mental development. Vitamin C also supports iron absorption. Iron is important for making hemoglobin, that carries oxygen to your cells, and maintains a healthy immune system. You will need extra iron for your growing baby and placenta, as well as to prevent iron-deficiency anemia, which can result in low birth weights and premature deliveries.

YIELDS: 1 QUART

1 cup iceberg lettuce
3 oranges, peeled
½ cup coconut milk

1. Blend iceberg and oranges until just combined.
2. Add coconut milk slowly while blending until desired consistency is reached.

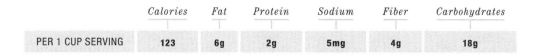

	Calories	Fat	Protein	Sodium	Fiber	Carbohydrates
PER 1 CUP SERVING	123	6g	2g	5mg	4g	18g

VITAMIN C

Oranges are well known for their immunity-building power, and rightfully so! Eating at least one orange a day can help expectant mothers stay healthy and strong throughout their pregnancy. You can thank the rich beta-carotenes and the vitamin C. An orange is a definite for health and longevity.

Splendid Citrus

Helps boost energy levels

Booming with the strong flavors of pineapple, orange, grapefruit, lemon, and lime, this sweet and tart smoothie will liven your senses. In addition, pineapple contains the enzyme bromelain, which has been said to help soften your cervix, which may stimulate your uterus and, toward the end of your pregnancy, may help induce labor.

YIELDS: 1 QUART

2 large kale leaves

1 cup pineapple, peeled and cubed

1 large orange or 2 small oranges, peeled

1 grapefruit, peeled

½ lemon, peeled

½ lime, peeled

1. Combine kale and all fruits in a blender in the order listed.
2. Blend until desired consistency is reached.

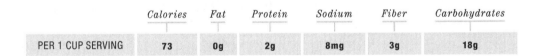

	Calories	*Fat*	*Protein*	*Sodium*	*Fiber*	*Carbohydrates*
PER 1 CUP SERVING	73	0g	2g	8mg	3g	18g

FEED YOUR BRAIN!

With 4 servings of fruit and 2 servings of vegetables, the vitamin and mineral benefits of this smoothie are obvious, but this citrusy green mix is also especially high in iron and folate. Necessary for optimal brain function, folate is especially important for pregnant and nursing women.

Coconut Craziness

Adding the flesh of the coconut and the coconut milk to this smoothie results in a sweet flavor that complements the iceberg nicely. This smoothie will make you crave coconuts like crazy!

1 cup iceberg lettuce
Flesh of 2 coconuts
1 cup coconut milk

1. Combine iceberg, coconut flesh, and ½ cup coconut milk in a blender, and blend.
2. Add remaining coconut milk while blending until desired texture is achieved.

	Calories	Fat	Protein	Sodium	Fiber	Carbohydrates
PER 1 CUP SERVING	172	15g	2g	9mg	1g	10g

Smoothies

Strawberry Start

Good for your baby's bones and development

If you love strawberries, you'll be happy to enjoy one of your favorite fruits while also fulfilling your daily requirement for an entire serving of greens. In addition, strawberries contain folate, which is important for the prevention of spina bifida. Consider buying organically grown strawberries to avoid exposure to synthetic pesticides.

YIELDS: 3–4 CUPS

½ cup dandelion greens

2 pints strawberries

1 cup vanilla soymilk

1 tablespoon agave nectar, to taste (optional)

1. Add dandelion greens, strawberries, and ½ cup soymilk to a blender and blend until combined.
2. Slowly add remaining ½ cup soymilk while blending until desired consistency is achieved.
3. Stop blending periodically to check for desired sweetness, and, if desired, drizzle in agave nectar until desired sweetness is achieved.

	Calories	Fat	Protein	Sodium	Fiber	Carbohydrates
PER 1 CUP SERVING	85	1g	3g	31mg	4g	17g

STRAWBERRIES FOR SIGHT

Rich in the antioxidants that give them their vibrant red color, this sweet berry is also rich in vitamins A, C, D, and E; B vitamins; and folate which are the most important vitamins to consume during your pregnancy for development, especially to support your baby's eyes.

Luscious Lemon-Lime

Good for strengthening your immune system

The tartness of the lemons and limes in this smoothie is cooled off with the crisp romaine and sweet agave nectar. The kefir gives a creamy texture with protein and essential vitamins. It also contains probiotics that have been shown to boost immunity during pregnancy. This smoothie should be eaten with a protein and grain, such as eggs and toast.

YIELDS: 2–3 CUPS

1 cup romaine lettuce

2 lemons, peeled

2 limes, peeled

½ cup kefir

1 tablespoon agave nectar

1. Combine romaine, lemons, limes, and kefir and blend until thoroughly combined.
2. Add agave nectar slowly while blending, stopping periodically to taste, until desired sweetness and texture are achieved.

	Calories	Fat	Protein	Sodium	Fiber	Carbohydrates
PER 1 CUP SERVING	111	2g	3g	36mg	5g	17g

Smoothies

The Green Go-Getter

Good for pregnancy cravings

Packed with green spinach and apples, this creamy green smoothie will kick off your morning with a boost of essential amino acids, vitamins, minerals, and an absolutely amazing taste. Since it has been said that 10 percent of pregnant women crave green apples, this smoothie may come in handy.

1 cup spinach

2 green apples, peeled and cored

1 banana, peeled

1 cup purified water

1. Combine spinach, apples, and banana with ½ cup of water in a blender and blend until thoroughly combined.
2. Continue adding remaining water while blending until desired texture is achieved.

	Calories	Fat	Protein	Sodium	Fiber	Carbohydrates
PER 1 CUP SERVING	89	0g	1g	10mg	3g	23g

Pear Splendor

Good for your digestive system

Pears give this smoothie its unique sweetness and taste while the banana adds a sweet, smooth texture. The pectin in pears may also act as a diuretic and mild laxative, which will help regulate your bowel movements throughout pregnancy. In addition, the folate found in pears helps prevent neural tube defects, especially when consumed early during pregnancy.

YIELDS: 3 CUPS

1 cup spinach

2 pears, cored and peeled

1 banana, peeled

1 cup almond milk

1. Combine spinach, pears, banana, and ½ cup almond milk in a blender and blend until smooth.
2. While blending, continue to add remaining almond milk until desired texture is achieved.

	Calories	Fat	Protein	Sodium	Fiber	Carbohydrates
PER 1 CUP SERVING	136	1g	1g	59mg	5g	33g

A Sweet Beet Smoothie

Helps boost energy levels

This deep-purple treat gets its color from the vibrant beets and deep-colored radicchio. The combination of vitamins A, B, C, E, and K and the protein from the creamy Greek-style yogurt, helps boost energy levels. The vitamins help your metabolism work more efficiently and the protein helps balance your blood sugars and energy levels. This smoothie also can help boost your iron levels during your last trimester, which can be tricky when your blood volume increases even more and your baby begins to store minerals.

YIELDS: 2–3 CUPS

1 cup radicchio
3 cups sliced beets
1 cup Greek-style yogurt

1. Combine the radicchio, beets, and ½ cup Greek-style yogurt in a blender and blend to combine thoroughly.
2. While blending, add remaining ½ cup yogurt until desired texture is achieved.

	Calories	Fat	Protein	Sodium	Fiber	Carbohydrates
PER 1 CUP SERVING	157	0g	15g	211mg	6g	25g

Pleasantly Pear

Good for your baby's bones and development

With the variety of fruits coupled with the romaine lettuce, this smoothie packs a whopping amount of vitamins, minerals, and antioxidants—including vitamins A and C—that provide your body with unsurpassed nutrition to pass on to your baby.

1 cup romaine lettuce
2 pears, peeled and cored
1 apple, peeled and cored
1 banana, peeled
½ cup purified water

1. Combine romaine, pears, apple, banana, and ¼ cup water in a blender and blend thoroughly.
2. While blending, add remaining water until desired texture is achieved.

	Calories	Fat	Protein	Sodium	Fiber	Carbohydrates
PER 1 CUP SERVING	132	0g	1g	4mg	6g	35g

FIBER EFFECTS OF PEARS

Fiber helps keep your digestive tract functioning optimally. Why not enjoy a smoothie that packs a whopping amount of fiber from greens, pears, and apples? This delicious smoothie can get your digestive system working at its best during pregnancy, especially when you experience cravings caused by unbalanced blood sugars or constipation, common pregnancy side effects.

Ginger and Spice Make Everything Nice

Good for morning sickness

This smoothie is packed with the delicious sweet and spicy flavor of ginger and the amazingly powerful taste of cloves. The addition of ginger can ward off morning sickness, nausea, and vomiting. In addition, the combination of vitamin-rich baby greens and potassium-packed banana will help you maintain hydration when morning sickness is dehydrating you. You may want to start enjoying this smoothie during your first trimester.

YIELDS: 3–4 CUPS

1 large nodule ginger, peeled and sliced

¾ cup almond milk

1 teaspoon cloves

1 cup baby greens

1 banana, peeled

1. Combine the ginger slices and half of the almond milk in a blender and combine thoroughly.
2. Once ginger has thickened the almond milk, add the cloves, baby greens, and banana.
3. While blending, add remaining almond milk until desired texture is achieved.

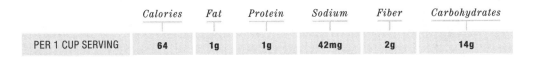

	Calories	Fat	Protein	Sodium	Fiber	Carbohydrates
PER 1 CUP SERVING	64	1g	1g	42mg	2g	14g

HARNESS THE POWER OF GINGER

Ayurvedic health practitioners use gingerroot as a treatment for an astounding number of ailments. By including the ginger with the greens and banana, the phytochemicals and antioxidants in this smoothie are powerful in boosting immunity for both you and your and baby.

Mango Madness

Good for healthy skin and hair

The color of this smoothie is vibrant, and the beta-carotene and vitamins A and E will help your skin look and feel fabulous during pregnancy. Dandelion greens add vitamin A, calcium, and iron, which support cell repair, perfect for keeping your skin looking its best.

YIELDS: 3–4 CUPS

½ **cup dandelion greens**
½ **cup romaine lettuce**
2 **mangos, peeled and pits removed**
1 **banana, peeled**
½ **cup purified water**

1. Combine dandelion greens, romaine, mangos, banana, and ¼ cup water in a blender and combine thoroughly.
2. While blending, add remaining water until desired texture is achieved.

	Calories	Fat	Protein	Sodium	Fiber	Carbohydrates
PER 1 CUP SERVING	130	1g	1g	12mg	4g	34g

Calming Cucumber

Your stress levels are bound to increase during pregnancy, but the light taste of cucumber and the powerfully fragrant mint combine with the deep green romaine in this delightfully smooth and refreshing smoothie to help you regain your footing. It can be the sweet end to your day.

1 cup romaine lettuce
2 cucumbers, peeled
¼ cup mint, chopped
1 cup purified water

1. Combine romaine, cucumbers, mint, and ½ cup water in a blender and combine thoroughly.
2. Add remaining water while blending until desired texture is achieved.

	Calories	Fat	Protein	Sodium	Fiber	Carbohydrates
PER 1 CUP SERVING	24	0g	1g	9mg	2g	4g

Splendid Melon

Good for your baby's bones and development

While endive is more commonly found in salads or as a garnish, this green is a wonderful base to this smoothie. The cantaloupe and honeydew melon add sweet nectar that will quench any need your body may have and they also add vitamin C, which will help your baby grow strong teeth and bones. In addition, endive provides an abundance of vitamin A to promote your baby's overall development.

YIELDS: 3–4 CUPS

1 cup endive, chopped

1 cantaloupe, peeled and
    seeds removed

1 honeydew, peeled and
    seeds removed

½ cup ice cubes (optional)

1. Combine endive, cantaloupe, and honeydew in a blender and blend thoroughly until desired texture is achieved.
2. If a thicker consistency is desired, ice can be added while blending until desired consistency is reached.

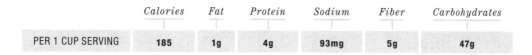

	Calories	Fat	Protein	Sodium	Fiber	Carbohydrates
PER 1 CUP SERVING	185	1g	4g	93mg	5g	47g

Tempting Tomato

Good for your baby's nervous system

The sweet yet tangy twist that results from the combination of the cabbage, tomatoes, celery, and peas is an inviting savory treat that can be enjoyed morning, noon, or night. It is recommended to have two servings of dark green leafy vegetables per day during pregnancy, so this smoothie gets you halfway there. In addition, the folic acid from the cabbage, tomatoes, and celery found in this smoothie help to ensure that your baby-to-be will have a strong, healthy nervous system.

YIELDS: 3–4 CUPS

1 cup cabbage
2 tomatoes, skin intact
1 stalk celery
½ cup sweet peas
½ cup purified water

1. Combine cabbage, tomatoes, celery, peas, and half of the water in a blender and blend until thoroughly combined.
2. Continue adding remaining water while blending until desired texture is achieved.

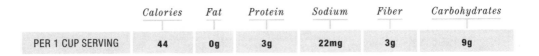

	Calories	Fat	Protein	Sodium	Fiber	Carbohydrates
PER 1 CUP SERVING	44	0g	3g	22mg	3g	9g

PASS THE PEAS, PLEASE

There's no veggie easier than the pea! Sweet and refreshing, you can serve them hot or munch on them cold. They require little prep time and taste great in a variety of dishes. This tiny veggie packs a punch in terms of all of the vitamins and nutrients it delivers. One cup of peas provides 50 percent of your daily value of vitamin K, which optimizes your baby's growth and development.

Super Celery

This combination of greens and rich vegetables offers a healthy dose of fiber; vitamins A, B, C, and K; and a wealth of minerals like iron and potassium. In addition, the presence of celery—traditionally used as a diuretic—can help you get rid of excess fluid, including the puffiness that can build up under your eyes and in your feet during pregnancy.

1 cup spinach
3 stalks celery
1 cucumber, peeled
1 carrot, peeled
1 cup purified water

1. Combine spinach, celery, cucumber, carrot, and ½ cup water in a blender and blend until thoroughly combined.
2. Continue adding remaining water as you blend until desired texture is achieved.

	Calories	Fat	Protein	Sodium	Fiber	Carbohydrates
PER 1 CUP SERVING	34	0g	1g	72mg	3g	7g

Smoothies

Very Veggie

Good for your baby's nervous system

If you're not in the mood for a huge bowl of salad, or if you're suffering from morning sickness, this Very Veggie smoothie can provide you and your baby with the same level of nutrition in much less time. Spinach acts as the green base to this smoothie, and the plentiful colors and tastes come from the addition of celery, carrots, tomato, green onion, and parsley, which are all good for your baby-to-be's nervous system.

YIELDS: 3–4 CUPS

1 cup spinach

2 stalks celery

2 carrots, peeled

1 tomato

1 green onion

1 small sprig parsley
   (optional)

1 cup purified water

1. Combine the spinach, celery, carrots, tomato, green onion, parsley (if desired), and ½ cup water in a blender and blend until combined thoroughly.
2. If necessary, continue adding remaining water while blending until desired texture is achieved.

	Calories	Fat	Protein	Sodium	Fiber	Carbohydrates
PER 1 CUP SERVING	32	0g	1g	62mg	2g	7g

THE POWER OF PARSLEY

That green garnish that arrives as a decoration on the side of your plate is not given the attention it deserves! This green leafy herb is rich in vitamins and minerals. In just one serving of this cleansing green, there are impressive amounts of vitamins K, C, and A, as well as iron and folate.

Go, Go, Garlic!

Good for strengthening your immune system

Yes, garlic is a great addition to your smoothie for a variety of reasons. One component of garlic contains allicin, a phytochemical that strengthens your immune system during pregnancy by fighting off free radicals in your body that can cause cell damage. Garlic can also be used to treat hypertension during pregnancy, which is a major concern in the third trimester. The bonus benefit of garlic is that if you eat large amounts of it during pregnancy, your baby may exhibit a preference for the flavor. In addition, the tomatoes and basil found in this recipe contain vitamin C, which acts as an antioxidant to help strengthen your and your baby-to-be's immune systems.

YIELDS: 2 CUPS

1 cup romaine lettuce

2 tomatoes

½ cup basil leaves

3 cloves garlic, crushed and left to sit for 1 hour

½ cup purified water (if necessary)

1. Combine romaine, tomatoes, basil, and garlic in a blender and combine thoroughly until all garlic is emulsified.
2. Add water while blending, if needed, until desired consistency is reached.

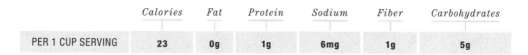

	Calories	Fat	Protein	Sodium	Fiber	Carbohydrates
PER 1 CUP SERVING	23	0g	1g	6mg	1g	5g

One Superb Herb

Good for your baby's nervous system

Although basil has become more and more common as a main ingredient in things like pesto and pasta sauce, this herb still doesn't get the attention it deserves for the health benefits it offers you and your baby-to-be. Basil provides vitamin K, vitamin A, manganese, and folate, all of which work together to strengthen your baby's immune system and support the growth of your baby's heart, lungs, kidneys, eyes, and bones.

YIELDS: 3–4 CUPS

1 cup iceberg lettuce

½ cup basil

1 cucumber, peeled

1 clove garlic

½ cup purified water

1. Combine the iceberg, basil, cucumber, and garlic in a blender with half of the water and blend until combined thoroughly.
2. If needed, continue adding remaining water while blending until desired texture is achieved.

	Calories	Fat	Protein	Sodium	Fiber	Carbohydrates
PER 1 CUP SERVING	14	0g	1g	5mg	1g	3g

Fresh Start

Good for morning sickness

This delicious blend of crisp watercress, refreshing melons, and zippy ginger deliver a taste combination that will refresh your body and mind while relieving your morning sickness.

YIELDS: 3–4 CUPS

1 cup watercress

2 cups watermelon, deseeded

½ cantaloupe, rind and seeds removed

½" ginger, peeled

1 cup caffeine-free raspberry tea

1. Combine watercress, watermelon, cantaloupe, ginger, and ½ cup tea in a blender and blend until thoroughly combined.
2. Add remaining ½ cup of tea as needed while blending until desired consistency is achieved.

	Calories	Fat	Protein	Sodium	Fiber	Carbohydrates
PER 1 CUP SERVING	38	0g	1g	20mg	1g	9g

Circulatory Smoothie

Good for fighting infections during pregnancy

One beautiful benefit of this blend is better circulation and reduced swelling in the legs—bye-bye, cankles! In addition, this smoothie works to fight infections ranging from the common cold to a bladder infection during pregnancy. The vitamin C in this smoothie can assist in healing your symptoms that follow infections by acting at an antioxidant to help your body fight back. Pregnancy stress can often put you at risk for infections, so this smoothie will help bring you back to yourself.

YIELDS: 3–4 CUPS

1 cup watercress

1 grapefruit, peeled

½ cantaloupe, rind and
   seeds removed

½ pineapple, peeled and
   cored

1 cup strawberries

1 cup caffeine-free
   raspberry tea

1. Combine watercress, grapefruit, cantaloupe, pineapple, strawberries, and ½ cup tea in a blender and blend until thoroughly combined.
2. Add remaining ½ cup tea as needed while blending until desired consistency is achieved.

	Calories	Fat	Protein	Sodium	Fiber	Carbohydrates
PER 1 CUP SERVING	112	0g	2g	17mg	2g	29g

Stomach Soother

Good for morning sickness

The majority of digestive problems that you may experience during pregnancy can be easily remedied with smoothies like this one due to the addition of ginger for morning sickness or an upset stomach. The comforting ginger will soothe your stomach while satisfying your taste buds.

YIELDS: 3–4 CUPS

1 cup watercress
3 apples, peeled and cored
1 banana, peeled
½" ginger, peeled
2 cups caffeine-free red raspberry tea

1. Combine watercress, apples, banana, ginger, and 1 cup of tea in a blender and blend until thoroughly combined.
2. Add remaining 1 cup of tea as needed while blending until desired consistency is achieved.

	Calories	Fat	Protein	Sodium	Fiber	Carbohydrates
PER 1 CUP SERVING	86	0g	1g	6mg	2g	22g

Good Morning Smoothie

Good for morning sickness

One of the major discomforts of pregnancy can be the queasiness, nausea, and vomiting brought on by almost anything. This smoothie recipe can be a perfect solution, whether you're an occasional or a constant sufferer of morning sickness. The ginger will alleviate your symptoms, while the vitamin C will give you a boost to get you back on your feet.

YIELDS: 3–4 CUPS

1 cup watercress
1 grapefruit, peeled
½ lemon, peeled
½" ginger, peeled
1 cup caffeine-free
    raspberry tea

1. Combine watercress, grapefruit, lemon, ginger, and ½ cup tea in a blender and blend until thoroughly combined.
2. Add remaining ½ cup of tea as needed while blending until desired consistency is achieved.

	Calories	Fat	Protein	Sodium	Fiber	Carbohydrates
PER 1 CUP SERVING	31	0g	1g	7mg	1g	8g

Creamy, Nutty, Sweet Smoothie

Good for pregnancy cravings

This sensational recipe delivers a delightfully creamy smoothie packed with protein, potassium, and omega-3s. It can satisfy your pregnancy cravings for sweets, creaminess, or nutty flavors!

YIELDS: 3–4 CUPS

¼ **cup almonds**

1 **tablespoon flaxseed**

2 **cups rice milk**

1 **cup watercress**

2 **bananas, peeled**

1. Combine almonds, flaxseed, and ½ cup rice milk in a blender and blend until completely emulsified and no bits of almonds remain.
2. Add watercress, bananas, and 1 cup of rice milk and blend until thoroughly combined.
3. Add remaining ½ cup of rice milk as needed while blending until desired consistency is achieved.

	Calories	Fat	Protein	Sodium	Fiber	Carbohydrates
PER 1 CUP SERVING	149	6g	3g	30mg	3g	22g

Smoothies

Peas for a Perfect Pregnancy

Good for your baby's nervous system

Although probably not the veggie that comes to mind when you think "superfood," peas are an excellent source of iron and folate—both important vitamins and minerals for promoting the best health in mom and a healthy nervous system for your baby!

1 cup arugula

1 cup sweet peas

2 stalks celery

1 cucumber, peeled

1 cup caffeine-free
   raspberry tea

1. Combine arugula, sweet peas, celery, cucumber, and ½ cup tea in a blender and blend until thoroughly combined.
2. Add remaining ½ cup of tea as needed while blending until desired consistency is achieved.

	Calories	Fat	Protein	Sodium	Fiber	Carbohydrates
PER 1 CUP SERVING	36	0g	2g	56mg	2g	7g

Berry Happy Mama

Good for pregnancy cravings

When Mama's happy, everyone's happy. Satisfying and refreshing ingredients combine here for a flavorful smoothie you can enjoy guilt-free. This smoothie provides both protein, found in kefir, and an abundance of fiber, found in berries and bananas. When protein and fiber are present, your blood sugars balance out and so does your hunger and energy levels. Cravings mostly occur when you don't choose foods with protein and fiber or go too long without eating. You'll be doing your body and baby good with this smoothie!

YIELDS: 3–4 CUPS

1 cup watercress
2 bananas, peeled
1 cup blueberries
1 cup strawberries
2 cups kefir

1. Combine watercress, bananas, berries, and 1 cup kefir in a blender and blend until thoroughly combined.
2. Add remaining 1 cup of kefir as needed while blending until desired consistency is achieved.

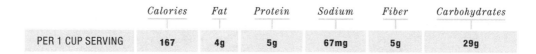

	Calories	Fat	Protein	Sodium	Fiber	Carbohydrates
PER 1 CUP SERVING	167	4g	5g	67mg	5g	29g

Crazy Carrot

Helps boost energy levels

If you think it is crazy that a green vegetable smoothie could be sweet, delicious, *and* increase your energy levels, think again! The powerhouse character of carrots gives you vitamins B, A, C, and K and fiber, which will be efficiently absorbed from choosing whole foods for your energy boost. However, the carrots you purchase make a difference. Buy organic carrots or fresh local carrots to avoid potential chlorine exposure.

YIELDS: 3–4 CUPS

1 cup romaine lettuce
3 carrots, peeled
1 banana, peeled
½ cup vanilla or plain almond milk

1. Combine romaine, carrots, banana, and ¼ cup almond milk in a blender and blend until thoroughly combined.
2. If needed, add remaining almond milk while blending until desired consistency is reached.

	Calories	Fat	Protein	Sodium	Fiber	Carbohydrates
PER 1 CUP SERVING	78	1g	1g	69mg	3g	18g

Sublime Lime

Good for strengthening your immune system

The tart taste of lime in this smoothie is balanced nicely with the addition of the sweet and thickening banana, which makes this smoothie a sweet treat that may give your face a reason to pucker up momentarily! It is common to crave limes and citrus during your pregnancy and this smoothie can also help boost both your and your baby-to-be's immune systems! There has been mention to avoid this fabulous fruit due to its acidity, however there is no evidence they are unsafe to consume during pregnancy. In fact, some pregnant women reported craving it throughout their pregnancy and you can also boost your vitamin C in one sip.

YIELDS: 3–4 CUPS

1 cup spinach
2 limes, peeled and
  deseeded
1 banana, peeled
½ cup purified water

1. Combine spinach, limes, and banana in a blender with ¼ cup water and blend until thoroughly combined.
2. If needed, add remaining water while blending until desired consistency is achieved.

	Calories	Fat	Protein	Sodium	Fiber	Carbohydrates
PER 1 CUP SERVING	51	0g	1g	10mg	2g	14g

The Pregnancy Helper

Good for morning sickness

When you start feeling like nine months is a long time, this smoothie is the perfect pick to calm your head and your stomach while pleasing your taste buds. Gingerroot's capabilities include alleviating symptoms associated with indigestion, nausea, and fever.

YIELDS: 3–4 CUPS

1 cup iceberg lettuce
1 apple, cored and peeled
1 banana, peeled
½"–1" gingerroot, peeled and sliced or chopped
1 cup vanilla almond milk

1. Combine iceberg, apple, banana, ginger, and ½ cup almond milk in a blender and blend until thoroughly combined.
2. If needed, add remaining almond milk while blending until desired texture is achieved.

	Calories	Fat	Protein	Sodium	Fiber	Carbohydrates
PER 1 CUP SERVING	103	1g	1g	54mg	3g	24g

A Bitter-Sweet Treat

Good for strengthening your immune system

The watercress, carrots, and sweet fruits in this recipe make for a tantalizing smoothie you won't soon forget! Watercress is a great source of vitamin C that helps keep both your and your baby-to-be's immune systems up to par.

YIELDS: 3–4 CUPS

1 cup watercress

3 carrots, peeled

2 apples, cored and peeled

1 banana, peeled

1 cup coconut milk

1. Combine watercress, carrots, apples, banana, and ½ cup coconut milk in a blender and blend until thoroughly combined.

2. If needed, add remaining ½ cup of coconut milk while blending until desired texture is achieved.

	Calories	Fat	Protein	Sodium	Fiber	Carbohydrates
PER 1 CUP SERVING	205	12g	2g	44mg	4g	25g

WATERCRESS

You may have heard of watercress, but never actually tried it. If that's the case, you'll be pleasantly surprised with this smoothie. With a delicious taste, this green (not a lettuce, but a green) is rich in disease-fighting properties that will keep your immune system, brain, blood, and bones running at optimal levels.

Green Gazpacho

Helps boost energy levels

This smoothie is modeled after gazpacho, a delightful cold soup prepared from a tomato base with onions, cucumber, bell pepper, and garlic. If you missed your vegetable servings for the day, this is the perfect smoothie for a nutrient and energy boost. Remember, you and your baby both need your veggies!

YIELDS: 3–4 CUPS

1 cup watercress

2 tomatoes

1 cucumber, peeled

1 stalk celery

½ red onion

½ green pepper

3 cloves garlic

1 small jalapeño (optional)

3 tablespoons red wine vinegar

2 tablespoons basil leaves, chopped

1 cup purified water, if needed

1. Combine all ingredients except the purified water in a blender and blend until thoroughly combined.
2. If needed, slowly add purified water while blending until desired texture is achieved.

	Calories	Fat	Protein	Sodium	Fiber	Carbohydrates
PER 1 CUP SERVING	34	0g	2g	18mg	2g	7g

Oh, Sweet Cabbage

Good for your baby's nervous system

As a delightfully sweet morning starter or equally enjoyable afternoon pick-me-up, this smoothie's combination of cabbage, carrots, and apples will have you wondering why you never considered cabbage a treat before. All fruits and vegetables, including cabbage, which is full of folate and antioxidants, allow your body to heal and grow, as well as help ensure that your baby's nervous system develops appropriately.

YIELDS: 3–4 CUPS

1 cup cabbage

3 carrots, peeled

1 apple, cored and peeled

1 cup purified water

1. Combine cabbage, carrots, and apple with ½ cup water in a blender and blend until thoroughly combined.

2. Add remaining ½ cup water slowly while blending until desired texture is achieved.

	Calories	Fat	Protein	Sodium	Fiber	Carbohydrates
PER 1 CUP SERVING	48	0g	1g	37mg	3g	12g

Savoy Smoothie

Helps boost energy levels

The strong beta-carotenes in this smoothie will help keep you energized and focused throughout the day. Whether you're looking for a great morning start or a quick and healthy lunch between doctor's appointments, this smoothie is a great go-to!

1 cup Savoy cabbage

1 beet, peeled (can be
   boiled or raw)

1 carrot, peeled

1 apple, cored and peeled

1 banana, peeled

1 cup vanilla soymilk

1. Combine the cabbage, beet, carrot, apple, and banana with ½ cup of the soymilk in a blender and blend until thoroughly combined.
2. Add remaining ½ cup of soymilk while blending until desired texture is achieved.

	Calories	Fat	Protein	Sodium	Fiber	Carbohydrates
PER 1 CUP SERVING	95	1g	3g	56mg	4g	20g

SAVOY AND VITAMIN K

Cabbage is packed with vitamin K, whose most well-known benefit is its large responsibility in blood clotting; however, it also plays an important role in the growth and development of your baby-to-be during pregnancy. By consuming just 1 cup of Savoy cabbage, you'll be getting more than 90 percent of your RDA of vitamin K. Your vitamin K needs do not increase during pregnancy, but you'll want to make sure you're receiving adequate amounts.

The Slump Bumper

Helps boost energy levels

You can't compare the energizing effects of the natural sugars (fructose) found in the sweet fruits and vegetables used in this recipe with the short-lived effects of energy drinks or junk foods that may contain chemicals and stimulants. This smoothie is a guilt-free natural energy booster that will keep you going even into your third trimester.

YIELDS: 3–4 CUPS

1 cup spinach
2 pears, cored and peeled
1 cup cherries, pitted
1 banana, peeled
2 cups almond milk

1. Combine spinach, pears, cherries, banana, and 1 cup of almond milk in a blender and blend until thoroughly combined.
2. Add remaining cup of almond milk while blending until desired texture is achieved.

	Calories	Fat	Protein	Sodium	Fiber	Carbohydrates
PER 1 CUP SERVING	149	2g	2g	82mg	5g	35g

Beet Booster

Good for your baby's nervous system

Beet greens and beets are not only delicious, they're especially good sources of folate. And this purple smoothie is not only attractive, it's an amazingly fresh way to sneak plenty of fruit and vegetable servings into your diet—and help boost your baby's forming nervous system. Don't be alarmed if you discover red or pink in your urine after drinking this smoothie, though. Ten to fourteen percent of the population have this experience.

YIELDS: 3–4 CUPS

1 cup beet greens

3 beets

1 banana, peeled

2 cups purified water

1. Combine beet greens, beets, banana, and 1 cup of water in a blender and blend until thoroughly combined.
2. Add remaining cup of water while blending until desired texture is achieved.

	Calories	Fat	Protein	Sodium	Fiber	Carbohydrates
PER 1 CUP SERVING	55	0g	2g	72mg	3g	13g

Berry, Berry Delicious

Good for fighting infections during pregnancy

The sweet tang of oranges, strawberries, and blueberries in this smoothie develops a deliciously refreshing treat that protects your body from bladder infections, which can be especially common when you're expecting. The berries in this smoothie are also good sources of fiber and can help your digestive system do its job well.

YIELDS: 3–4 CUPS

1 cup romaine lettuce
2 oranges, peeled
1 cup strawberries
1 cup blueberries
1 cup vanilla almond milk

1. Combine the romaine, oranges, berries, and ½ cup of almond milk in a blender and blend until thoroughly combined.
2. Add remaining ½ cup of almond milk while blending until desired texture is achieved.

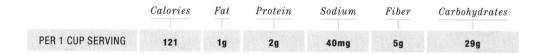

	Calories	Fat	Protein	Sodium	Fiber	Carbohydrates
PER 1 CUP SERVING	121	1g	2g	40mg	5g	29g

CITRIC ACID AND FLAVOR

Lemon, lime, and orange juices are commonly used in foods and drinks with the main purpose of enhancing the flavors of the main ingredient. A small amount of acidic citrus juice can add a depth to the flavors of fruits or vegetables, and the result in smoothies containing berries is an amplified sweetness of the berries' natural flavors.

Peachy Berry

Good for healthy skin and hair

If you love peaches and berries, combining them with the baby greens in this smoothie delivers sweet tastes with an incredible number of vitamins and nutrients. Vitamin A, C, and E can curb any damage to your skin caused by pregnancy stress and can also help smooth and firm skin and strengthen your hair. This smoothie can help repair damage to your hair or skin possibly caused by stress during pregnancy. Just peachy!

1 cup baby greens

2 peaches, pitted and peeled

1 cup strawberries

1 banana, peeled

½ tablespoon ginger, sliced
   or grated

Purified water, to taste
   (optional)

1. Add all ingredients to a blender and blend until thoroughly combined.
2. Add water if necessary while blending, if smoothie is too thick.

	Calories	Fat	Protein	Sodium	Fiber	Carbohydrates
PER 1 CUP SERVING	92	1g	2g	3mg	4g	23g

ORGANIC ALERT!

Peaches are an important fruit to purchase organic. Because of their thin flesh, they are more susceptible to the pesticides and preservatives used in the nonorganic growing process. Although more pricey than nonorganic varieties, buying organic peaches is important for your health and your soon-to-be baby's.

Apple-Ginger Delight

Good for pregnancy cravings

This satisfying smoothie can fulfill your sweet or salty cravings, and if you're not a huge fan of ginger, you can always vary the amount so it's more suitable to your palate. In addition, the protein and fiber combination found in this recipe is perfect for balancing your blood sugars and energy levels between meals.

YIELDS: 3–4 CUPS

1 cup romaine lettuce
2 apples, cored and peeled
½" nodule of gingerroot, peeled
½ cup Greek-style yogurt

1. Combine romaine, apples, ginger, and ¼ cup yogurt in a blender and blend until thoroughly combined.
2. Add remaining yogurt while blending until desired texture is achieved.

	Calories	Fat	Protein	Sodium	Fiber	Carbohydrates
PER 1 CUP SERVING	88	0g	4g	18mg	3g	19g

CRAVINGS FOR SWEETS

Every pregnant woman is familiar with the common craving. Cravings may vary from person to person—you may crave salty or sweet, for example. Either way, apples have been known to curb most cravings, and also create a feeling of fullness. When a craving hits, eat an apple with a full glass of water and wait 30 minutes. Chances are your craving will have subsided and you will have replaced a higher calorie option with a nutritious snack!

Smoothies

A Sweet Beet Treat

Good for pregnancy cravings

When you're looking for a sweet treat, beets are vitamin and nutrient packed. Beets are packed with fiber to balance blood sugars, energy levels, and cravings. In addition, it is recommended to have at least one source of vitamin A every other day, and beet greens are the perfect choice.

YIELDS: 3–4 CUPS

1 cup beet greens

3 beets

1 banana, peeled

1 cup almond milk

½ cup ice cubes (optional)

1. Combine beet greens, beets, banana, and ½ cup almond milk in a blender container and blend until thoroughly combined.
2. Add remaining almond milk and ice (if desired) while blending until desired texture is achieved.

	Calories	Fat	Protein	Sodium	Fiber	Carbohydrates
PER 1 CUP SERVING	77	1g	2g	107mg	3g	17g

BEET GREENS

While the actual beets are what have the reputation for being sweet, nutritious, delicious little veggies, the roots and greens of the beet are also edible and highly nutritious. Packed with calcium, potassium, and vitamins A and C, the roots and leaves of these powerful deep-purple veggies are a healthy addition to your diet during pregnancy.

Cool Cucumber Melon

Helps boost energy levels

The mix of romaine, mint, cucumbers, and honeydew in this recipe combine beautifully to develop one crisp smoothie. The way cucumbers help you feel good and put you in a good mood from their abundance of B vitamins is good enough reason to turn the blender on. B vitamins are known to be associated with energy levels, especially during the change of seasons, not to mention, they help your baby to grow and develop.

YIELDS: 3–4 CUPS

1 cup romaine lettuce

1 sprig mint leaves

3 cucumbers, peeled

½ honeydew melon,
    peeled, seeds removed

½ cup kefir

1. In a blender, combine romaine and mint leaves followed by the cucumbers, melon, and ¼ cup kefir and blend until thoroughly combined.
2. Add remaining kefir while blending until desired texture is achieved.

	Calories	Fat	Protein	Sodium	Fiber	Carbohydrates
PER 1 CUP SERVING	86	1g	3g	43mg	3g	17g

A Berry Delicious End to the Day

Good for pregnancy cravings

When the sweetness of a berry smoothie sounds just perfect, treat yourself to this home-made version that offers both health benefits and the peace of mind from knowing exactly how it's made. And with so many ingredients in commercially made products, this smoothie will help you be a role model of clean eating for years to come.

YIELDS: 3–4 CUPS

1 cup iceberg lettuce

1 pint strawberries

1 pint blueberries

1 banana, peeled

½ cup vanilla almond milk

½ cup ice cubes (optional)

1. Combine iceberg, strawberries, blueberries, banana, and almond milk in a blender until thoroughly combined.
2. Add optional ice cubes while blending until desired texture is achieved.

	Calories	Fat	Protein	Sodium	Fiber	Carbohydrates
PER 1 CUP SERVING	111	1g	2g	22mg	5g	27g

BERRIES AND THE BLADDER

Although many people consider them just tasty fruits, berries are well-known superfoods that can improve health and prevent illness. In addition to contributing to strong heart health, blueberries and cranberries promote bladder health by acting as a guard against E. coli bacteria, which is the culprit in urinary tract infections. Pregnant women are more vulnerable to urinary tract infections—especially between weeks six and twenty-four—because the urinary tract is changing and the uterus sits directly on top of the bladder. This can cause a blockage during drainage, which can lead to an infection.

Wacky Watermelon

Good for morning sickness

Watermelon's amazing taste isn't the only great thing about this fruit! Watermelon has been shown to ease heartburn and reduce swelling in pregnant women, and morning sickness and dehydration may also be alleviated due to its 92 percent water content. Lastly, the minerals it contains can help prevent third-trimester muscle cramps. Drink up!

YIELDS: 3–4 CUPS

1 cup iceberg lettuce

½ sprig mint leaves

2 cups watermelon

1 cucumber, peeled

Purified water, to taste
    (optional)

1. Combine the iceberg, mint, watermelon, and cucumber in a blender and blend until thoroughly combined.
2. Add water, if necessary, while blending until desired texture is achieved.

	Calories	Fat	Protein	Sodium	Fiber	Carbohydrates
PER 1 CUP SERVING	32	0g	1g	4mg	1g	7g

Chocolatey Dream

Good for pregnancy cravings

Ahhhh, chocolate! This smoothie has the perfect blend of ingredients to satisfy any chocolate craving. In addition, flavonoids—antioxidants that produce the color properties in plants and have anti-inflammatory benefits for the body—are responsible for the well-known benefits of cocoa and are capable of relaxing your veins. This can lower your blood pressure, a common problem in late pregnancy.

YIELDS: 3–4 CUPS

1 cup watercress

2 tablespoons raw powdered cocoa

2 bananas, peeled

2 cups almond milk

1. In a blender, combine the watercress and cocoa powder, followed by the bananas and 1 cup of the almond milk and blend until thoroughly combined.
2. Add remaining cup of almond milk while blending until desired texture is achieved.

	Calories	Fat	Protein	Sodium	Fiber	Carbohydrates
PER 1 CUP SERVING	104	2g	2g	80mg	3g	23g

CHOCOLATE IS HEALTHY?

Chocolate has been determined to be beneficial in the daily diet! Now, don't take this as a go-ahead to dive into that huge bag of M&M's. Powdered, unprocessed cocoa is the chocolate shown to provide the most benefits. Although the candy bar alternative may seem more gratifying, the sugar content, trans fats, and milk products may be the reason they haven't yet been labeled superfoods and have been shown to cause more harm to our health. However, if you're choosing cacao or unprocessed cocoa to enjoy during your pregnancy you can receive the benefits it has to offer.

The Joy of Almonds

Good for pregnancy cravings

If that Almond Joy candy is what satisfies your sweet tooth, this smoothie is for you. Packed with the flavors of almonds and coconut, this creamy smoothie will surely become one of your favorites! The protein and fiber from almonds provide a tool for subsiding pregnancy cravings, but the delicious flavor combination of coconut, almonds, and banana might make your cravings go away on its own!

YIELDS: 3–4 CUPS

½ cup almonds
2 cups fresh coconut milk
   (not canned)
1 cup romaine lettuce
Flesh of 2 mature coconuts
1 banana

1. Combine the almonds and ½ cup of coconut milk in a blender and emulsify until most remnants of the almonds have been liquefied, adding more liquid as needed.
2. Add the romaine, coconut flesh, banana, and 1 cup of coconut milk and blend until thoroughly combined.
3. Add remaining ½ cup of coconut milk, if needed, while blending until desired texture is achieved.

	Calories	Fat	Protein	Sodium	Fiber	Carbohydrates
PER 1 CUP SERVING	650	46g	13g	56mg	21g	44g

Pumpkin Spice

Good for your digestive system

Pumpkins are good for pregnant women. How? They can relieve abdominal cramps during pregnancy when they are cooked. They can also eliminate eczema, edema, and relieve the common condition of constipation in women who are expecting. Their composition of vitamins A and C and fiber make pumpkins perfect for the job.

YIELDS: 3–4 CUPS

½ cup pumpkin, cubed or diced

1 cup vanilla soymilk

1 cup romaine lettuce

1 teaspoon cloves

1 tablespoon ginger, grated

½ cup Greek-style yogurt

1. Combine pumpkin and ½ cup soymilk in a blender until completely emulsified.
2. Add romaine, cloves, ginger, and yogurt and blend until thoroughly combined.
3. If needed, add remaining soymilk while blending until desired consistency is achieved.

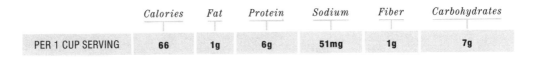

	Calories	Fat	Protein	Sodium	Fiber	Carbohydrates
PER 1 CUP SERVING	66	1g	6g	51mg	1g	7g

THE POWER OF PUMPKIN

Rich in vitamins and nutrients, this beta-carotene–rich squash contains a surprising amount of the nutrition you need throughout your pregnancy. Pumpkin contains more than 140 percent of your daily value of vitamin A in just ½ cup. By consuming pumpkin with ginger, yogurt, and soymilk in this smoothie, you'll be getting a protein-packed, vitamin-rich treat that will satisfy your need for pumpkin pie any time of year.

Sweet Potato Pie

Good for your baby's nervous system

Eating for two can be a nerve-wracking responsibility; however, the flavors and nutrition from this smoothie will help build your confidence. Sweet potatoes contain carotenoids, which are converted to vitamin A, which are so important for your baby-to-be's circulatory, respiratory, and central nervous systems. The bonus of this smoothie is that the sweet potatoes and spinach in this recipe provide you with a great source of vitamin C, folate, and fiber.

YIELDS: 3–4 CUPS

2 sweet potatoes, peeled and cut for blender's ability

2 cups vanilla soymilk

1 teaspoon cloves

½"–1" knob of ginger

1 cup spinach

1. Combine the sweet potatoes with 1 cup vanilla soymilk in a blender and blend until sweet potato is completely emulsified.
2. Add cloves, ginger, and spinach and blend until thoroughly combined.
3. Add remaining 1 cup of soymilk while blending until desired texture is achieved.

	Calories	Fat	Protein	Sodium	Fiber	Carbohydrates
PER 1 CUP SERVING	111	2g	4g	91mg	3g	19g

Coconut Cream Smoothie

Good for pregnancy cravings

This recipe blends the star ingredients of coconut cream pie, coconut, and banana, in a healthy smoothie. Consuming coconut during pregnancy can help keep away constipation and heartburn and the protein from the Greek yogurt and the fiber from the banana and coconut will take care of cravings by slowing your digestion and increasing your satiety.

YIELDS: 3–4 CUPS

1 cup romaine lettuce

Flesh of 2 mature coconuts

1 tablespoon lemon juice

1 banana, peeled

¼" ginger, peeled

½ cup almond milk

½ cup Greek-style yogurt

1. Combine romaine, coconut flesh, lemon juice, banana, ginger, and almond milk in a blender until thoroughly combined.
2. Add the yogurt while blending until desired texture is achieved.

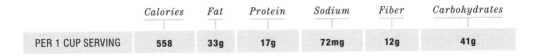

	Calories	Fat	Protein	Sodium	Fiber	Carbohydrates
PER 1 CUP SERVING	558	33g	17g	72mg	12g	41g

Sinful Strawberry Cream

Good for your baby's bones and development

Rich, sweet, and creamy, this recipe will simultaneously satisfy your sweet tooth and your daily value of important vitamins and minerals. Folate is high in these berries and can help prevent birth defects and premature birth. Since strawberries have been placed on the Environmental Working Group's "Dirty Dozen" list (a list that provides the top food items found to be highest in pesticides), you're advised to buy organic strawberries, especially while pregnant.

YIELDS: 3–4 CUPS

1 cup spinach
2 pints strawberries
1 banana, peeled
1 cup kefir

1. Combine spinach, strawberries, banana, and ½ cup kefir in a blender container and blend until thoroughly combined.
2. Add remaining ½ cup kefir while blending until desired texture is achieved.

	Calories	Fat	Protein	Sodium	Fiber	Carbohydrates
PER 1 CUP SERVING	126	3g	4g	39mg	5g	24g

KEFIR VERSUS MILK

If you've never indulged in this delicious milk alternative, now may be the perfect time to try it out and receive more benefits for you and your baby. Kefir contains a plethora of vitamins, beneficial probiotic bacteria, and rich enzymes that promote healthy growth, optimize digestion, and fight illness. The best part is that almost every grocery store that carries milk products will carry kefir, so the switch is as easy as walking further down the aisle.

Raspberry Delight

Good for your baby's nervous system

This smoothie packs protein, iron, folate, and B vitamins galore that will support your baby-to-be's nervous system. In addition, the fiber content in this recipe will put you well on your way to meet the recommended amount of 25–30 grams of fiber every day.

YIELDS: 3–4 CUPS

1 cup iceberg lettuce

2 pints raspberries

1 banana, peeled

½ cup rice milk

½ cup Greek-style yogurt

1. Combine iceberg, raspberries, banana, and rice milk in a blender and blend until thoroughly combined.
2. Add Greek-style yogurt while blending until desired texture is achieved.

	Calories	Fat	Protein	Sodium	Fiber	Carbohydrates
PER 1 CUP SERVING	141	1g	5g	28mg	11g	30g

Banana Nut Blend

Good for pregnancy cravings

The protein content of walnuts and fiber from bananas will ward off cravings by balancing your blood sugars, and the best thing is that you can enjoy this smoothie in the morning or night. Why? Because walnuts can bring calmness to a restless night of sleep by boosting your body's melatonin levels. They can even help you maintain a healthy milk supply during breastfeeding, so continue to enjoy this smoothie once your little one arrives.

YIELDS: 3–4 CUPS

¼ cup walnuts

1 cup vanilla almond milk

1 cup romaine lettuce

2 bananas, peeled

1. Combine walnuts and ½ cup almond milk in a blender and blend until walnuts are completely emulsified.
2. Add romaine, bananas, and remaining ½ cup almond milk while blending until desired texture is achieved.

	Calories	Fat	Protein	Sodium	Fiber	Carbohydrates
PER 1 CUP SERVING	99	6g	2g	39mg	2g	12g

WALNUTS AND ANTIOXIDANTS

When you think of antioxidant-rich foods, walnuts probably aren't your first thought, but just ¼ cup of walnuts carries almost 100 percent of your daily value of omega-3 fatty acids, and is loaded with monounsaturated fats. Of the tree nuts, walnuts, chestnuts, and pecans carry the highest amounts of antioxidants, which can prevent illness and reverse oxidative damage done by free radicals. Antioxidants are especially important during pregnancy for protecting you and your baby.

Blueberry Supreme

Good for strengthening your immune system

Blueberries take center stage in this antioxidant-packed, day-brightening recipe! These little fruits are one of the top ten foods to eat during pregnancy as they can help both you and your baby receive three times the amount of antioxidants, which protect your immune system from any free radicals that could potentially cause harm or illnesses.

YIELDS: 3–4 CUPS

1 cup iceberg lettuce

2 pints blueberries

1 banana, peeled

½ cup rice milk

1. Combine iceberg, blueberries, banana, and ¼ cup rice milk in a blender and blend until thoroughly combined.
2. Add remaining rice milk while blending until desired texture is achieved.

	Calories	Fat	Protein	Sodium	Fiber	Carbohydrates
PER 1 CUP SERVING	128	1g	2g	16mg	5g	32g

Berry Bananas

Helps boost energy levels

This smoothie is packed with fiber and protein, which makes it a complete snack and perfect for an afternoon pick-me-up. So, make this smoothie before going out for your afternoon errands. You'll be satisfied until dinner.

YIELDS: 4–6 CUPS

1 cup romaine lettuce
1 pint blueberries
1 pint raspberries
2 pints strawberries
2 bananas, peeled
1 cup vanilla almond milk
1 cup Greek-style yogurt

1. Combine romaine, berries, bananas, and milk in a blender and blend until thoroughly combined.
2. Add Greek-style yogurt while blending until desired texture is achieved.

	Calories	Fat	Protein	Sodium	Fiber	Carbohydrates
PER 1 CUP SERVING	230	2g	9g	66mg	11g	49g

Go Nuts for Chocolate!

Good for pregnancy cravings

You may only think of eating nuts by the handful, but nuts are actually the perfect food to add to your smoothies. Almonds are one of the most nutritious nuts, because they are high in calcium, B vitamins, and vitamin E, all of which are crucial for a healthy baby. In addition, the protein from the almonds and the fiber from the banana in this recipe will help you beat your cravings. Talk about a win-win!

YIELDS: 3–4 CUPS

¼ cup almonds

1 cup vanilla almond milk

2 tablespoons raw powdered cocoa

1 cup watercress

1 banana, peeled

1 tablespoon agave nectar (optional)

1. Combine almonds and ½ cup almond milk in a blender and blend until almonds are completely emulsified.

2. Add cocoa, followed by the watercress, banana, nectar, and remaining ½ cup almond milk while blending until desired texture is achieved.

	Calories	Fat	Protein	Sodium	Fiber	Carbohydrates
PER 1 CUP SERVING	143	7g	4g	56mg	4g	19g

Mango Supreme

Good for your baby's bones and development

Mangos and bananas make one sweet combination, and with the amazing amounts of vitamins, minerals, and phytochemicals you get from blending them with rich greens, this smoothie is the perfect combination of delightful taste and sound nutrition. The calcium and magnesium of mangos can relax your muscles and relieve the day's stress, and the vitamin A and vitamin C are crucial in building your baby's bones and supporting each developmental stage throughout pregnancy.

YIELDS: 3–4 CUPS

1 cup iceberg lettuce

2 mangos, peeled and pits
   removed

1 banana, peeled

2 cups purified water

1. Combine iceberg, mangos, banana, and 1 cup of water in a blender and blend until thoroughly combined.

2. Add remaining cup of water while blending until desired texture is achieved.

	Calories	Fat	Protein	Sodium	Fiber	Carbohydrates
PER 1 CUP SERVING	96	0g	1g	7mg	3g	25g

Just Peachy

Good for your baby's nervous system

Peaches can offer a sweet nectar taste to almost anything. They also offer you a smoothie full of folic acid, vitamin A, vitamin C, vitamin E, and potassium . . . all of which will help your baby-to-be's nervous system develop correctly. This smoothie would go perfectly with a protein—such as ¼ cup of nuts or a Greek yogurt—during snack time.

YIELDS: 3–4 CUPS

1 cup romaine lettuce

3 peaches, pitted (peel removed, optional)

1 banana

½ cup water

1. Combine romaine, peaches, banana, and ¼ cup of water in a blender and blend until thoroughly combined.
2. Add remaining ¼ cup of water while blending until desired texture is achieved.

	Calories	Fat	Protein	Sodium	Fiber	Carbohydrates
PER 1 CUP SERVING	72	0g	1g	2mg	3g	18g

A Daring Pearing

Good for fighting infections during pregnancy

Because pears aren't in season year round, the frozen option is available at almost any grocery store, and will make equally delicious green smoothies. Pears provide your taste buds with a delicious mouthful of fiber and vitamin C that will help keep you healthy throughout your pregnancy.

YIELDS: 3–4 CUPS

1 cup spinach

3 pears, peeled and cored

1 banana, peeled

1 cup purified water

1. Combine spinach, pears, banana, and ½ cup water in a blender and blend until thoroughly combined.
2. Add remaining ½ cup water while blending until desired texture is achieved.

	Calories	Fat	Protein	Sodium	Fiber	Carbohydrates
PER 1 CUP SERVING	105	0g	1g	9mg	5g	28g

Great Granny Smith

Good for morning sickness

Up to 90 percent of pregnant women experience the nausea and vomiting that accompanies morning sickness and many have found relief with a tart Granny Smith apple. In addition, this smoothie brings great satisfaction to your sour cravings, especially if you're craving a sour apple candy.

YIELDS: 3–4 CUPS

1 cup spinach

3 Granny Smith apples,
   peeled and cored

2 bananas

2 cups purified water

1. Combine spinach, apples, bananas, and 1 cup of water in a blender and blend until thoroughly combined.
2. Add remaining cup of water while blending until desired texture is achieved.

	Calories	Fat	Protein	Sodium	Fiber	Carbohydrates
PER 1 CUP SERVING	112	0g	1g	9mg	3g	29g

Veggie Variety

Good for your baby's bones and development

With variety comes a beneficial array of the important vitamins and nutrients that keep your baby growing and your body running like an efficient machine. The combination of the spinach, tomato, cucumber, and celery in this recipe pack it full of vitamins A and C, calcium, folate, and potassium—all of which are necessary for a healthy pregnancy and to support your baby's bones and development.

YIELDS: 3–4 CUPS

1 cup spinach
1 tomato
1 cucumber, peeled
2 stalks celery
1 clove garlic
1 cup purified water

1. Combine spinach, tomato, cucumber, celery, garlic, and ½ cup of purified water in a blender and blend until thoroughly combined.
2. Add remaining ½ cup water while blending until desired texture is achieved.

	Calories	Fat	Protein	Sodium	Fiber	Carbohydrates
PER 1 CUP SERVING	18	0g	1g	26mg	1g	3g

CUCUMBERS

Store your unwashed cucumbers in your refrigerator for up to ten days. Wash them just before using. Leftover cucumbers can be refrigerated again; just tightly wrap them in plastic and they will keep for up to five days.

A Spicy Assortment

Variety is the spice of life and this savory smoothie offers a salty, spicy, and amazingly delicious combination of vegetables. It could also be a reasonable replacement for a Bloody Mary during your pregnancy.

1 cup arugula
2 carrots, peeled
1 zucchini
1 stalk celery
½ jalapeño, or to taste
1 clove garlic
1 cup purified water

1. Combine arugula, carrots, zucchini, celery, jalapeño, garlic, and ½ cup water in a blender and blend until thoroughly combined.
2. Add remaining water while blending until desired texture is achieved.

	Calories	Fat	Protein	Sodium	Fiber	Carbohydrates
PER 1 CUP SERVING	35	0g	2g	49mg	2g	8g

Awesome Asparagus

Rich in vitamins K, A, and C; the B-complex vitamins; folate; and a variety of minerals like iron and zinc, the benefits of asparagus surpass those of many other veggies. Introducing one cup of asparagus to your day promotes heart health, digestive health, and regularity, and satisfies a daily serving requirement of vegetables.

YIELDS: 3–4 CUPS

1 cup romaine lettuce

1 cup asparagus

1 green onion

1 stalk celery

1 clove garlic

2 cups purified water

Juice of ½ lemon

1. Combine romaine, asparagus, onion, celery, garlic, and 1 cup of purified water in a blender and blend until thoroughly combined.
2. Add remaining cup of water and lemon juice while blending until desired texture and taste are achieved.

	Calories	Fat	Protein	Sodium	Fiber	Carbohydrates
PER 1 CUP SERVING	12	0g	1g	3mg	1g	3g

Blazing Broccoli

Good for your baby's bones and development

It's likely that you grew up hearing, "You need to finish your broccoli," and you'll likely be saying it as your baby grows up. The truth is that broccoli is one of the most powerfully packed superfoods you can find! Known for being a good source of calcium, this veggie is also packed with vitamin C, folate, and vitamin B_6, all of which will help your baby-to-be develop strong bones and a healthy growth pattern.

YIELDS: 3–4 CUPS

1 cup spinach

1 cup broccoli

1 carrot, peeled

1 green pepper, cored

½ lime, peeled

2 cups purified water

1. Combine spinach, broccoli, carrot, pepper, lime, and 1 cup of purified water in a blender and blend until thoroughly combined.
2. Add remaining 1 cup water while blending until desired texture is achieved.

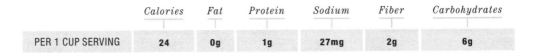

	Calories	Fat	Protein	Sodium	Fiber	Carbohydrates
PER 1 CUP SERVING	24	0g	1g	27mg	2g	6g

Kale Carrot Combo

Good for your baby's bones and development

Since it's packed with vitamins K, A, C, and B_6; calcium; iron; and folate, kale is a green that provides you with many benefits during your pregnancy. The calcium and vitamins A and C support your baby's bones and the vitamins K, A, and C support your baby's overall development. Lastly, folate supports the proper development of your baby's nervous system. And, unlike spinach or chard, kale doesn't contain oxalic acid, which can prevent the body from absorbing calcium. In fact, the calcium in kale is more easily absorbed than that in milk, and if you're breastfeeding, eating kale can even help to increase your milk supply.

YIELDS: 3–4 CUPS

2 kale leaves
4 carrots, peeled
1 apple, cored and peeled
1 banana, peeled
2 cups purified water

1. Combine kale leaves, carrots, apple, banana, and 1 cup purified water in a blender and blend until thoroughly combined.

2. Add remaining 1 cup of water while blending until desired texture is achieved.

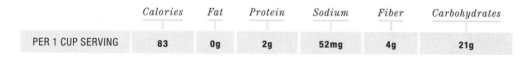

	Calories	Fat	Protein	Sodium	Fiber	Carbohydrates
PER 1 CUP SERVING	83	0g	2g	52mg	4g	21g

Fantastic Fennel

Good for fighting infections during pregnancy

Although it can be found in almost every grocery store's produce section, people rarely purchase fennel or prepare it at home, which is a shame! The vitamins and minerals in this veggie make it a must-have, and the taste is amazingly unique. Fennel is a good source of vitamin C, which helps repair tissues and fight infections, such as bladder infections, during pregnancy. However, vitamin C can also help your baby's cartilage, tendons, skin, and bones grow strong and healthy. You'll need about 80 mg of vitamin C per day and this recipe provides approximately 30mg.

YIELDS: 3–4 CUPS

1 cup romaine lettuce
2 bulbs fennel
1 cucumber, peeled
1 carrot, peeled
1 stalk celery
2 cups purified water

1. Combine romaine, fennel, cucumber, carrot, celery, and 1 cup of purified water in a blender and blend until thoroughly combined.

2. Add remaining 1 cup of water while blending until desired texture is achieved.

	Calories	Fat	Protein	Sodium	Fiber	Carbohydrates
PER 1 CUP SERVING	52	0g	2g	84mg	5g	12g

Zippy Zucchini

Helps boost energy levels

Zucchini is well known for being a blank canvas in terms of flavor, and the addition of savory ingredients along with the spicy arugula in this recipe delivers a smoothie with a bite. During the nine months of your pregnancy, zucchini is important to incorporate for its B complex that will help with your energy levels and moods.

YIELDS: 3–4 CUPS

1 cup arugula
2 zucchini
1 stalk celery
1 tomato
1 clove garlic
2 cups purified water

1. Combine arugula, zucchini, celery, tomato, garlic, and 1 cup water in a blender and blend until thoroughly combined.
2. Add remaining 1 cup of water while blending until desired texture is achieved.

	Calories	Fat	Protein	Sodium	Fiber	Carbohydrates
PER 1 CUP SERVING	25	0g	2g	23mg	2g	5g

Sweet and Savory Beet

Beets and their greens are filled with antioxidants and vitamins. Beet greens are often over-looked, but they are a great source of vitamins A and C and folate and are a perfect addition to your smoothie to help support your baby's bones, development, and nervous system.

YIELDS: 3–4 CUPS

1 cup beet greens

2 beets

2 carrots, peeled

1 cucumber, peeled

2 cups purified water

1. Combine beet greens, beets, carrots, cucumber, and 1 cup water in a blender and blend until thoroughly combined.
2. Add remaining 1 cup water while blending until desired texture is achieved.

	Calories	Fat	Protein	Sodium	Fiber	Carbohydrates
PER 1 CUP SERVING	38	0g	1g	78mg	3g	8g

BEET COLORS

Beets come in many colors, from deep red to orange. They also can be white. The Chioggia beet is called a candy cane beet because it has red and white rings. Small or medium beets are more tender than larger ones. Beets can be enjoyed on their own or flavored with some butter, salt, and pepper for a simple side dish if you're craving something simple.

The Green Bloody Mary

Good for pregnancy cravings

The alcoholic Bloody Mary may be tempting, but this green version of the Bloody Mary has all of the necessary ingredients to help you and your baby feel great! If you're craving an alcoholic beverage, serving this juice in a fancy glass could help you feel a part of the party. However, the watercress also will help prevent you from developing iron-deficiency anemia, which can be more common among pregnant women. It also assists in the process of carrying oxygen to other cells for you and your baby.

YIELDS: 3–4 CUPS

1 cup watercress

2 tomatoes

2 stalks celery

½ lemon, peeled

1 tablespoon horseradish

½ teaspoon cayenne
   pepper (optional)

1 cup purified water

1. Combine watercress, tomatoes, celery, lemon, horseradish, and cayenne with ½ cup purified water in a blender and blend until thoroughly combined.
2. Add remaining ½ cup water while blending until desired texture is achieved.

	Calories	Fat	Protein	Sodium	Fiber	Carbohydrates
PER 1 CUP SERVING	19	0g	1g	36mg	1g	4g

Cabbage Carrot

Good for your baby's bones and development

Cabbage is one of those important veggies that makes an appearance only on special holidays, and then it's usually not prepared or paired in the most nutritious ways. This recipe blends it with tasty green celery to provide a great source of folate that supports your baby's development and nervous system and can prevent neurological birth defects. Cabbage also provides a good amount of vitamin C and calcium that support your baby's bone growth.

YIELDS: 3–4 CUPS

1 cup green cabbage

3 carrots, peeled

2 stalks celery

1" nodule ginger, peeled
   and sliced

2 cups purified water

1. Combine cabbage, carrots, celery, ginger, and 1 cup water in a blender and blend until thoroughly combined.
2. Add remaining 1 cup water while blending until desired texture is achieved.

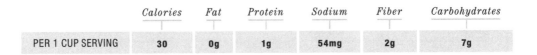

	Calories	Fat	Protein	Sodium	Fiber	Carbohydrates
PER 1 CUP SERVING	30	0g	1g	54mg	2g	7g

Powerful Pepper Trio

Helps boost energy levels

The vibrant colors of the peppers used in this recipe show their powerful vitamin-rich content, which makes for a delicious and nutritious treat. This smoothie's mix of spicy arugula, peppers, and garlic combine for a savory treat you can enjoy anytime—especially if you're looking for an energy boost throughout your pregnancy! The vitamin pack of A, C, K, B_6, plus the folate and calcium can certainly awaken your cells, leaving you feeling energized.

YIELDS: 3–4 CUPS

1 cup arugula

1 red pepper, cored

1 green pepper, cored

1 yellow pepper, cored

1 clove garlic

2 cups purified water

1. Combine arugula, peppers, garlic, and 1 cup of water in a blender and blend until thoroughly combined.
2. Add remaining 1 cup water while blending until desired texture is achieved.

	Calories	Fat	Protein	Sodium	Fiber	Carbohydrates
PER 1 CUP SERVING	29	0g	1g	6mg	2g	7g

Smoothies

Great Garlic

Helps boosts energy levels

Garlic is the main attraction in this smoothie that could potentially reduce fatigue during pregnancy. Just one small clove of garlic helps promote a strong heart—which is needed when you're pumping double the amount of blood—and makes almost anything taste absolutely delightful.

1 cup spinach
1 stalk celery
1 tomato
3 cloves garlic
2 cups purified water

1. Combine spinach, celery, tomato, garlic, and 1 cup water in a blender and blend until thoroughly combined.
2. Add remaining 1 cup water, if needed, while blending until desired texture is achieved.

	Calories	Fat	Protein	Sodium	Fiber	Carbohydrates
PER 1 CUP SERVING	12	0g	1g	18mg	1g	3g

Savory Celery Celebration

Good for healthy skin and hair

This may surprise you, but celery is a powerful ingredient and skin-beautifying food that will have you feeling and looking fabulous during your pregnancy. Celery is rich in vitamin C, which is needed to make the collagen that helps keep your skin strong, and the mineral silica, an element that helps your skin return to its pre-pregnancy condition once you have the baby.

YIELDS: 3–4 CUPS

1 cup watercress

3 stalks celery

1 cucumber, peeled

1 clove garlic

1 cup purified water

1. Combine watercress, celery, cucumber, garlic, and ½ cup water in a blender and blend until thoroughly combined.
2. Add remaining ½ cup water while blending until desired texture is achieved.

	Calories	Fat	Protein	Sodium	Fiber	Carbohydrates
PER 1 CUP SERVING	13	0g	1g	30mg	1g	2g

Savory Squash Surprise

When you take a look at the color of this smoothie, you'll see the vibrant colors of the veggies, and thus their valuable nutrition. The bright-green spinach, yellow squash, and orange carrot combine for an aesthetic, palate-pleasing smoothie. There are many nutrients in this smoothie that will benefit you throughout your entire pregnancy, such as vitamins A and C, folate, and fiber. However, it will also help you get beautiful skin and hair with its abundance of vitamins A and C.

YIELDS: 3–4 CUPS

1 cup spinach
½ butternut squash, peeled, deseeded, and cubed
1 carrot, peeled
2 cloves garlic
2 cups purified water

1. Combine spinach, squash, carrot, garlic, and 1 cup of water in a blender and blend until thoroughly combined.
2. Add remaining 1 cup of water while blending until desired texture is achieved.

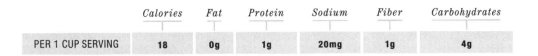

	Calories	Fat	Protein	Sodium	Fiber	Carbohydrates
PER 1 CUP SERVING	18	0g	1g	20mg	1g	4g

Turnip Temptation

Good for your baby's nervous system

Rich in nutrition, the turnip—this rarely enjoyed root vegetable—is a great addition to any meal, especially when you think about its folate content. The daily requirement for pregnant women is 600mcg and this smoothie contains about 60mcg.

1 cup romaine lettuce

2 turnips, peeled and cut best for blender's ability

2 carrots, peeled

2 stalks celery

2 cups purified water

1. Combine romaine, turnips, carrots, celery, and 1 cup water in a blender and blend until thoroughly combined.
2. Add remaining 1 cup of water while blending until desired texture is achieved.

	Calories	Fat	Protein	Sodium	Fiber	Carbohydrates
PER 1 CUP SERVING	35	0g	1g	81mg	3g	8g

Vitamin C Smoothie

Good for strengthening your immune system

Immunity and health are never as important as when you're pregnant. And not only does the vitamin C found in this recipe make for an important addition to your diet for its strong immunity-building power, this vitamin also benefits you by providing optimal brain functioning. That means better mental clarity, improved focus, and an overall feeling of awareness that is far superior to the mental fuzziness commonly referred to as "pregnancy brain."

YIELDS: 3–4 CUPS

1 cup watercress
2 tangerines, peeled
½ grapefruit, peeled
½ pineapple, peeled and
    cored
½ cantaloupe, rind and
    seeds removed
1 cup red raspberry tea

1. Combine watercress, tangerines, grapefruit, pineapple, and cantaloupe in a blender and blend until thoroughly combined.
2. Add tea as needed while blending until desired consistency is achieved.

	Calories	Fat	Protein	Sodium	Fiber	Carbohydrates
PER 1 CUP SERVING	114	0g	2g	18mg	2g	29g

Imperative Iron

Helps boost energy levels

Pregnant women require 27mg of iron per day (as opposed to 18mg when not pregnant) and, thanks to the broccoli in this recipe, this smoothie is full of it! Iron is responsible for making hemoglobin that carries oxygen to your cells. Because many women are iron deficient prior to becoming pregnant, their needs are even higher and the risks associated with iron deficiencies are more severe. Preterm delivery, low birth weight, infant mortality, and decreased energy levels are all risks of iron deficiencies in pregnancy. So skip the chips and drink down this savory, satisfying smoothie!

YIELDS: 3–4 CUPS

1 cup spinach
2 carrots, peeled
½ cup broccoli spears
½ cup asparagus spears
1 clove garlic
2 cups caffeine-free red
   raspberry tea

1. Combine spinach, carrots, broccoli, asparagus, garlic, and 1 cup of tea in a blender and blend until thoroughly combined.
2. Add remaining 1 cup of tea as needed while blending until desired consistency is achieved.

	Calories	Fat	Protein	Sodium	Fiber	Carbohydrates
PER 1 CUP SERVING	23	0g	1g	34mg	2g	5g

Ginger Melon Stress Meltaway

Although pregnancy is an amazing experience of excitement and anticipation, stress and moodiness can sometimes make it seem unbearable. Calm your nerves while quieting cravings with this delicious combination of watercress, melons, citrus, and ginger.

1 cup watercress

½ cantaloupe, rind and
   seeds removed

½ honeydew, rind and
   seeds removed

1 tangerine, peeled

½" ginger, peeled

1 cup red raspberry tea

1. Combine watercress, cantaloupe, honeydew, tangerine, and ginger in a blender and blend until thoroughly combined.
2. Add tea as needed while blending until desired consistency is achieved.

	Calories	Fat	Protein	Sodium	Fiber	Carbohydrates
PER 1 CUP SERVING	94	0g	2g	45mg	2g	24g

Cabbage, Broccoli, and Celery

Good for fighting infections during pregnancy

The discomforts of pregnancy aren't limited to nausea. Bacterial infections resulting from hormonal fluctuations can be worsened by diet and can lead to discomfort. Fortunately, the cabbage, broccoli, and celery found in this recipe are rich in vitamin C that helps combat infections and will keep you feeling great for all three trimesters!

YIELDS: 3–4 CUPS

1 cup cabbage

½ cup broccoli

½ cup cauliflower

1 stalk celery

2 cups caffeine-free
   raspberry tea

1. Combine cabbage, broccoli, cauliflower, celery, and 1 cup of tea in a blender and blend until thoroughly combined.
2. Add remaining 1 cup of tea as needed while blending until desired consistency is achieved.

	Calories	Fat	Protein	Sodium	Fiber	Carbohydrates
PER 1 CUP SERVING	19	0g	1g	29mg	2g	4g

Raspberry Immune System Smoothie

Good for strengthening your immune system

Protect your body and your baby from illness by packing in the vitamin C found in the oranges, pineapple, lemon, and lime in this recipe. Not only does this amazing vitamin promote health and immunity, it can alleviate stress and improve mental stability and happiness.

YIELDS: 3–4 CUPS

1 cup watercress

2 oranges, peeled

½ pineapple, peeled and cored

½ lemon, peeled

½ lime, peeled

1 cup red raspberry tea

1. Combine watercress, oranges, pineapple, lemon, and lime in a blender and blend until thoroughly combined.

2. Add tea as needed while blending until desired consistency is achieved.

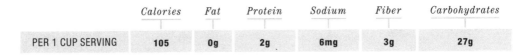

	Calories	Fat	Protein	Sodium	Fiber	Carbohydrates
PER 1 CUP SERVING	105	0g	2g	6mg	3g	27g

Moodiness Manipulator

Forget all of the nay-sayers who call pregnancy moodiness "crazy." Forty weeks is a long time, and the hormone fluctuations you're experiencing don't necessarily help you maintain a cool, calm, and collected composure all the time. Indulging in this delicious treat will lift your mood with its pack of vitamins C, A, and K; calcium; and the B-complex group. Preventing vitamin deficiencies is the most effective way to balance the possible symptoms from your hormone fluctuations during pregnancy.

YIELDS: 3–4 CUPS

1 cup watercress

½ cantaloupe, rind and
    seeds removed

½ lemon, peeled

½" ginger, peeled

1½ cups caffeine-free
    raspberry tea

1. Combine watercress, cantaloupe, lemon, ginger, and ¾ cup of the tea in a blender and blend until thoroughly combined.
2. Add remaining ¾ cup of tea as needed while blending until desired consistency is achieved.

	Calories	Fat	Protein	Sodium	Fiber	Carbohydrates
PER 1 CUP SERVING	27	0g	1g	17mg	1g	7g

NUTRITION FOR STABILITY

Creating life requires a lot of energy, and because your growing baby is depending on you for vitamins and minerals, deficiencies can leave you fatigued. Provide your body with all of the necessary nutrients to prevent common symptoms associated with deficiencies. You can improve your pregnancy experience with a diet rich in leafy greens and vibrant fruits and veggies.

Pleasurable Pregnancy Smoothie

Pregnancy is an opportunity to give your body the pristine treatment it deserves. Treat yourself to this delicious smoothie throughout your nine months and savor the feeling of optimal health that you'll get from the drinking down a glass full of vitamins C and A, and calcium. It's good health at its most delicious!

YIELDS: 3–4 CUPS

1 cup watercress

2 red Gala apples, peeled and cored

1 cup cranberries

¼" ginger, peeled

2 cups caffeine-free raspberry tea

1. Combine watercress, apples, cranberries, ginger, and 1 cup of tea in a blender and blend until thoroughly combined.
2. Add remaining 1 cup of tea as needed while blending until desired consistency is achieved.

	Calories	Fat	Protein	Sodium	Fiber	Carbohydrates
PER 1 CUP SERVING	51	0g	1g	6mg	2g	14g

PAMPER YOURSELF

Whether this is your first pregnancy or the next in a long line of lovable little ones, your pregnancy is a time that requires special attention. The hustle and bustle of everyday life can leave you run down and overwhelmed, and being pregnant can add to exhaustion and lack of focus on yourself. Take the time to spend quiet and quality time on yourself without distraction or stress. Meditation, light exercise, and quality nutrition can be the keys to a pampered pregnancy and provide happiness for all!

Savory Spinach

Good for your baby's bones and development

The benefits of iron are outstanding, and are even greater in pregnancy. Satisfy your nutritional needs and daily requirements—and help your baby-to-be grow and develop—with this smoothie recipe that combines iron-packed spinach with sweet red peppers, vitamin-packed broccoli, and spicy garlic that will keep energy flowing to all of your cells.

YIELDS: 3–4 CUPS

1 cup spinach
½ **red bell pepper, cored, ribs intact**
½ **cup broccoli spears**
1 clove garlic
2 cups caffeine-free red raspberry tea

1. Combine spinach, red pepper, broccoli, garlic, and 1 cup of tea in a blender and blend until thoroughly combined.
2. Add remaining 1 cup of tea as needed while blending until desired consistency is achieved.

	Calories	Fat	Protein	Sodium	Fiber	Carbohydrates
PER 1 CUP SERVING	15	0g	1g	17mg	1g	3g

Maternity Medley

This delicious smoothie recipe combines sweet fruits and luscious watercress with the zing of ginger to provide an abundance of important vitamins and minerals, such as vitamins A, C, K, and B complex, for your pregnancy. It will also sweeten your day—and what's better than that?

1 cup watercress
½ mango, peeled and
   deseeded
½ pineapple, peeled and
   cored
2 tangerines, peeled
¼" ginger, peeled
1 cup red raspberry tea

1. Combine watercress, mango, pineapple, tangerines, ginger, and ½ cup of tea in a blender and blend until thoroughly combined.
2. Add remaining ½ cup of tea as needed while blending until desired consistency is achieved.

	Calories	Fat	Protein	Sodium	Fiber	Carbohydrates
PER 1 CUP SERVING	98	0g	1g	7mg	1g	25g

MAKE CALORIES COUNT IN PREGNANCY

Although many women strive for complete nutrition while also appreciating the increase in caloric requirements suggested in pregnancy, some fear excess troublesome weight gain. In order to ensure that your nutrition and your weight gain are ideal for your pregnancy, make every calorie count! Empty-calorie foods like fried foods and sugary treats deliver empty nutrition for your body and your baby, and lead to excessive sodium, sugar, and fat intake, which will result in stubborn post-baby pounds.

Cran-Energy Smoothie

Helps boost energy levels

The blend of berries, melon, and vanilla found in this smoothie downplays the subtle taste of spinach, creating a deliciously sweet and tart smoothie that provides vitamins A, C, and K; magnesium; iron; and phytonutrients—plant components that protect your body from damage —and gives your cells a boost! In addition, the kefir provides protein to help you sustain those increased energy levels.

YIELDS: 3–4 CUPS

1 cup spinach

2 cups cranberries

1 cup cantaloupe, rind and seeds removed

Pulp of ½ vanilla bean

1 cup kefir

1. Combine spinach, cranberries, cantaloupe, vanilla pulp, and ½ cup kefir in a blender and blend until thoroughly combined.
2. Add remaining ½ cup of kefir as needed while blending until desired consistency is achieved.

	Calories	Fat	Protein	Sodium	Fiber	Carbohydrates
PER 1 CUP SERVING	78	2g	3g	44mg	4g	14g

Baby, Be Happy

This simple recipe makes a deliciously sweet veggie smoothie you're sure to enjoy. Here, the iron-rich spinach and peas combine with vitamin-rich carrots for a splendid creation that will satisfy your increasing iron needs.

YIELDS: 3–4 CUPS

1 cup spinach

1 cup sweet peas

3 carrots, peeled

2 cups caffeine-free red raspberry tea

1. Combine spinach, peas, carrots, and 1 cup of tea in a blender and blend until thoroughly combined.
2. Add remaining 1 cup of tea as needed while blending until desired consistency is achieved.

	Calories	Fat	Protein	Sodium	Fiber	Carbohydrates
PER 1 CUP SERVING	46	0g	2g	76mg	3g	9g

Folate-Filled Fruit Smoothie

The sweet blend of fruits and vibrant vegetables in this recipe make for one splendid smoothie that's packed with vitamins and minerals, such as vitamins C, A, K, E, and B complex; folate; iron; calcium; and potassium. This power-packed smoothie will help ensure that you feel your best through all three trimesters—and it's delicious too!

YIELDS: 3–4 CUPS

1 cup spinach

2 carrots, peeled

2 red Gala apples, peeled and cored

1 banana, peeled

2 cups caffeine-free red raspberry tea

1. Combine spinach, carrots, apples, banana, and 1 cup of tea in a blender and blend until thoroughly combined.
2. Add remaining 1 cup of tea as needed while blending until desired consistency is achieved.

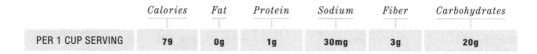

	Calories	Fat	Protein	Sodium	Fiber	Carbohydrates
PER 1 CUP SERVING	79	0g	1g	30mg	3g	20g

IMPORTANCE OF FOLATE IN PREGNANCY

Among the important vitamins and minerals found to prevent birth defects, one of the most well known is folate. Studies have shown that ideal levels of folate in pregnancy reduce or remedy the chance of neural and spinal-tube defects. You can take a prenatal vitamin that includes folate, but what about natural sources? Eating a diet rich in deep leafy greens and vibrant green vegetables can provide a great amount of folate naturally.

Veggies for Vitamins

This delicious savory blend of spicy arugula, tomato, cucumber, celery, onion, and garlic combines with natural tea to give your body an amazing amount of vitamins and minerals, such as vitamins A, C, and K; iron; and calcium. These are particularly important for your baby-to-be's bones and the development of his heart, muscles, and eyes.

YIELDS: 3–4 CUPS

1 cup arugula

1 tomato

1 cucumber, peeled

1 stalk celery

1 green onion

1 clove garlic

2 cups caffeine-free red raspberry tea

1. Combine arugula, tomato, cucumber, celery, onion, garlic, and 1 cup of tea in a blender and blend until thoroughly combined.

2. Add remaining 1 cup of tea as needed while blending until desired consistency is achieved.

	Calories	Fat	Protein	Sodium	Fiber	Carbohydrates
PER 1 CUP SERVING	17	0g	1g	15mg	1g	3g

Refreshing Raspberry Blend

Helps boost energy levels

Raspberries offer a tangy sweet taste that is heightened by the sweet pineapple and sour lemon in this recipe. Simple, quick, and delicious, this smoothie will be a favorite go-to when you're in need of a delicious snack in little time. The fiber from watercress, raspberries, and pineapple paired with protein from kefir will boost your energy levels throughout your pregnancy and keep you feeling your best!

YIELDS: 3–4 CUPS

1 cup watercress
1 cup raspberries
½ pineapple, peeled and cored
½ lemon, peeled
1½ cups kefir

1. Combine watercress, raspberries, pineapple, lemon, and ¾ cup of kefir in a blender and blend until thoroughly combined.
2. Add remaining ¾ cup of kefir as needed while blending until desired consistency is achieved.

	Calories	Fat	Protein	Sodium	Fiber	Carbohydrates
PER 1 CUP SERVING	136	3g	4g	52mg	3g	25g

Pregnant Pomegranate Smoothie

Since these delicious fruits and vegetables are packed with vitamins C, K, and B complex; potassium; and magnesium that all promote health and fight illness, this recipe is a tasty way to feel great throughout your pregnancy. And if getting into a pomegranate seems like too much work, know that the seeds you'll find inside are well worth the effort due to their high amounts of antioxidant that will fight off any free radicals attempting to cause damage to your cells and lower your immune system.

YIELDS: 3–4 CUPS

1 cup iceberg lettuce

2 cups pomegranate pips (seeds)

1 orange, peeled

1 banana, peeled

1 cup purified water

1. Combine iceberg, pomegranate, orange, banana, and ½ cup water in a blender and blend until thoroughly combined.
2. Add remaining ½ cup water as needed while blending until desired consistency is achieved.

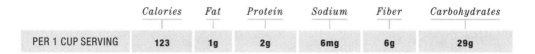

	Calories	Fat	Protein	Sodium	Fiber	Carbohydrates
PER 1 CUP SERVING	123	1g	2g	6mg	6g	29g

Beta-Carotene Cantaloupe Smoothie

The vibrant orange color of cantaloupe is from the abundant levels of beta-carotene, which is known for providing health benefits that are necessary for developing your baby's heart, lungs, kidneys, eyes, and bones. More than just a sweet treat, this smoothie provides a wide variety of vitamins and minerals—such as vitamin C, magnesium, and potassium—that work hard to prevent illness and disease by repairing your tissues and cells and keeping your body hydrated.

YIELDS: 3–4 CUPS

1 cup watercress
½ cantaloupe, rind and seeds removed
1 apple, peeled and cored
1 banana, peeled
¼" ginger, peeled
1 cup purified water

1. Combine watercress, cantaloupe, apple, banana, ginger, and ½ cup water in a blender and blend until thoroughly combined.
2. Add remaining ½ cup water as needed while blending until desired consistency is achieved.

	Calories	Fat	Protein	Sodium	Fiber	Carbohydrates
PER 1 CUP SERVING	70	0g	1g	16mg	2g	18g

Blackberry Delight

Good for strengthening your immune system

Delicious blackberries are made even more tasty with the addition of lemon and ginger in this recipe. But, in addition to great taste, this smoothie packs a healthy dose of much-needed vitamins and minerals—such as vitamins A, C, and K; potassium; and magnesium, that help strengthen your and your baby's immune systems—and is rich and satisfying with the addition of protein-packed yogurt.

YIELDS: 3–4 CUPS

1 cup watercress
2 pints blackberries
1 banana, peeled
½ lemon, peeled
½" ginger, peeled
1 cup Greek-style yogurt

1. Combine watercress, blackberries, banana, lemon, ginger, and ½ cup of yogurt in a blender and blend until thoroughly combined.
2. Add remaining ½ cup yogurt as needed while blending until desired consistency is achieved.

	Calories	Fat	Protein	Sodium	Fiber	Carbohydrates
PER 1 CUP SERVING	125	1g	8g	29mg	9g	25g

Romaine Pineapple Smoothie

Vitamins K and C, beta-carotene, potassium, folate, and protein are rich in this delicious smoothie. A one-stop shop for many of your fruit and vegetable servings, this delicious recipe satisfies your sweet tooth and your pregnancy dietary needs.

YIELDS: 3–4 CUPS

1 cup romaine lettuce

1 cup pineapple, peeled and cored

1 pint strawberries

1 banana, peeled

1 cup Greek-style yogurt

1. Combine romaine, pineapple, strawberries, banana, and ½ cup yogurt in a blender and blend until thoroughly combined.
2. Add remaining ½ cup yogurt as needed while blending until desired consistency is achieved.

	Calories	Fat	Protein	Sodium	Fiber	Carbohydrates
PER 1 CUP SERVING	108	0g	7g	26mg	3g	21g

Berry and Banana Smoothie

The crisp taste of iceberg lettuce is beautifully balanced with the addition of blackberries, citrus, bananas, and yogurt for a flavor combination that will make you enjoy eating better for your health. The calcium and vitamins A and C found in this smoothie are perfect for building your baby's bones and developing her organs, such as the heart, lungs, kidneys, and eyes.

YIELDS: 3–4 CUPS

1 cup iceberg lettuce
1 pint blackberries
1 cup pineapple, peeled and cored
2 bananas, peeled
1 cup Greek-style yogurt

1. Combine iceberg, blackberries, pineapple, bananas, and ½ cup yogurt in a blender and blend until thoroughly combined.
2. Add remaining ½ cup yogurt as needed while blending until desired consistency is achieved.

	Calories	Fat	Protein	Sodium	Fiber	Carbohydrates
PER 1 CUP SERVING	137	1g	8g	27mg	6g	29g

MAGNESIUM FOR BONE HEALTH

The magnesium in blackberries can do amazing things for respiratory relief, but that's not all it's good for! Magnesium plays an important role in the absorption of calcium, and a diet rich in this powerful mineral ensures strong bones for you and your baby.

A Grape Way to Bone Health

Good for your baby's bones and development

The sweetness of this smoothie just can't be beat! This recipe provides abundant vitamins, such as vitamins A, C, K, and B complex, and minerals such as calcium with the added benefit of an amazingly refreshing taste. These vitamins and minerals not only help your baby develop properly, they also will help your skin and energy levels throughout your pregnancy.

YIELDS: 3–4 CUPS

1 cup watercress
2 cups red grapes
2 pears, cored
1 banana, peeled
1 cup purified water

1. Combine watercress, grapes, pears, banana, and ½ cup of water in a blender and blend until thoroughly combined.
2. Add remaining ½ cup of water as needed while blending until desired consistency is achieved.

	Calories	Fat	Protein	Sodium	Fiber	Carbohydrates
PER 1 CUP SERVING	131	0g	1g	7mg	4g	34g

Smoothies

Vitamin C Pack

This vitamin C–packed recipe is a delicious blend of grapefruit, pineapple, and orange, intensified by the addition of ginger and iron and vitamin K-rich spinach. These ingredients will help during pregnancy by supporting the growth and development of your baby. Though vitamin K is often thought of for its role in the normal clotting of your blood, it is one of the most important vitamins for a healthy pregnancy. The presence of vitamin C also assists in growth and development, because it is necessary for the body to make collagen, which helps make your baby's cartilage, tendons, bones, and skin.

YIELDS: 3–4 CUPS

1 cup spinach
1 grapefruit, peeled
1 cup pineapple, peeled
and cored
1 orange, peeled
½" ginger, peeled
1 cup purified water

1. Combine spinach, grapefruit, pineapple, orange, ginger, and ½ cup water in a blender and blend until thoroughly combined.
2. Add remaining ½ cup water as needed while blending until desired consistency is achieved.

	Calories	Fat	Protein	Sodium	Fiber	Carbohydrates
PER 1 CUP SERVING	62	0g	1g	8mg	2g	16g

BANANA SMOOTHIES

Bananas make a tasty base to a variety of smoothies because their low water content makes them natural thickening agents. You can go fruity by mixing in some raspberries and blueberries for A Berry Great Morning, or blend a rich treat with almonds in the Creamy, Nutty, Sweet Smoothie. See recipes in Chapter 3.

MINT SMOOTHIES

The smell of mint is definitely refreshing, though that's not the only benefit of adding it to your smoothies. It also helps with digestion and nausea. If you want a nice minty treat, go ahead and blend a Calming Cucumber or A Cool Blend for Pregnancy. See recipes in Chapter 3.

BEET JUICE

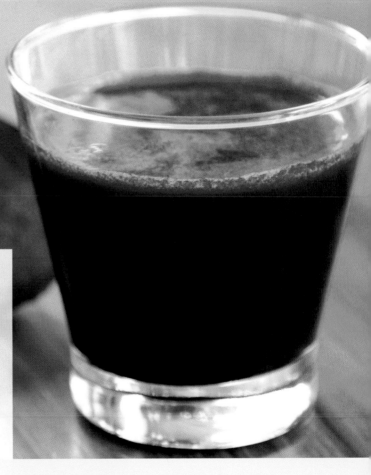

Besides making one tasty juice, beets are also great as a source of folic acid. You can mix and match your beet juice with fruits and vegetables to please your particular palate. Try a veggie-heavy mix with the Carrot, Cucumber, and Beet, or go a bit sweeter with the Apple Beeter. See recipes in Chapter 4.

MELON JUICE

The electrolytes and high water content of melons will keep your energy levels up during pregnancy and may even help alleviate morning sickness. If you prefer to keep it simple, try them on their own with Watermelon Straight Up and Cantaloupe Straight Up, or bring those flavors together in a refreshing glass of Super Melon. See recipes in Chapter 4.

MANGO JUICE

The tropical taste of mango juice is a great way to brighten up any day. Start things off on the right foot with the Rise and Shine recipe that marries that wonderful mango flavor with pineapple, peach, and banana. Then you can keep things upbeat and exotic later in the day with a glass of Mango Kiwifruit or Tropical Cucumber. See recipes in Chapter 4.

SPINACH SMOOTHIES

You don't need a salad bowl to get your fill of nutritious greens. Instead, try blending together smoothies that deliver all the amazing benefits of spinach with a variety of different flavors. Mix in some fruit with the Green Go-Getter or Great Granny Smith, or get the full salad-bar experience by combining spinach, celery, carrots, tomato, and onion in the Very Veggie. See recipes in Chapter 3.

CARROT AND APPLE JUICE

Carrots and apples make a tasty combination. This bright juice combo packs in vitamins A and C, and works nicely with additional flavors. Spice it up a bit with the Ginger Carrot Apple recipe, or go green by adding in some leafy vegetables for a glass of Carrot Kale. See recipes in Chapter 4.

PINEAPPLE JUICE

If you're having any digestive troubles during your pregnancy, pineapples may be your answer. Bromelain, an enzyme found in the fruit, is known to help with digestion. And with options like Pineapple Greets Papaya, Peach Pineapple, and Pineapple Plum Punch, your digestive aid will taste delicious! See recipes in Chapter 4.

A Cool Blend for Pregnancy

Helps boost energy levels

Maintaining eating patterns that optimize sugar levels to balance your energy is easy with this delicious blend. The combination of ingredients makes a refreshing treat that will keep you going when you need a boost.

1 cup watercress

1 stalk celery

1 cucumber, peeled

2 pears, cored

2 tablespoons mint

1 cup Greek-style yogurt

1. Combine watercress, celery, cucumber, pears, mint, and ½ cup yogurt in a blender and blend until thoroughly combined.
2. Add remaining ½ cup yogurt as needed while blending until desired consistency is achieved.

	Calories	Fat	Protein	Sodium	Fiber	Carbohydrates
PER 1 CUP SERVING	94	0g	7g	38mg	4g	18g

Cherry Vanilla Treat

Move over, ice cream! This delicious smoothie will have you wondering, "Is this really good for me?" Although the delicious flavors of cherry and vanilla take center stage, the vitamin and mineral content of all the ingredients (including the spinach) will do your baby a world of good. This smoothie is full of vitamins C, A, and K and calcium, which will help your baby's heart, lungs, kidneys, eyes, and bones develop—and it's delicious to boot!

YIELDS: 3–4 CUPS

1 cup spinach
2 cups cherries, pitted
1 apple, peeled and cored
Pulp of 1 vanilla bean
½" ginger, peeled
2 cups purified water

1. Combine spinach, cherries, apple, vanilla, ginger, and 1 cup water in a blender and blend until thoroughly combined.
2. Add remaining 1 cup of water as needed while blending until desired consistency is achieved.

	Calories	Fat	Protein	Sodium	Fiber	Carbohydrates
PER 1 CUP SERVING	73	0g	1g	9mg	2g	18g

Watermelon and Watercress Smoothie

If your diet and lifestyle leave you feeling in need of refreshment and vitality, this smoothie is for you. Hydrating melon and citrus combine with rich greens to provide a revitalizing lift in energy levels throughout your pregnancy. The water content found in watermelon will hydrate and supply your body with vitamins A, C, and B_6 that will boost your energy for the day. Dehydration can lead to exhaustion and fatigue, so drink up!

YIELDS: 3–4 CUPS

1 cup watercress
2 cups watermelon
1 cup pineapple, peeled
 and cored
1 cup kefir

1. Combine watercress, watermelon, pineapple, and ¾ cup kefir in a blender and blend until thoroughly combined.
2. Add remaining ¼ cup kefir as needed while blending until desired consistency is achieved.

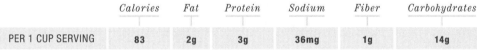

	Calories	Fat	Protein	Sodium	Fiber	Carbohydrates
PER 1 CUP SERVING	83	2g	3g	36mg	1g	14g

THE BODY'S NEED FOR WATER

Cravings, fatigue, lack of focus, and derailed bodily functions can all result from not getting adequate water. The minimum recommended water intake is eight 8-ounce glasses of water daily, but those who exercise require even more. In addition to the water added while blending, the fruits and vegetable in this smoothie deliver one tasty way to increase your hydration.

Apple Celery Smoothie

Helps boost energy levels

The fruits and greens in this smoothie provide natural sugars and carbohydrates that will supply your body with efficient fuel to keep you feeling great. In addition, the celery in this recipe regulates fluid levels in your body to support hydration, which will keep you feeling energized, and the apples provide an adequate amount of fiber that will help slow your digestion, balance blood sugars, and sustain energy levels.

YIELDS: 3–4 CUPS

1 cup romaine lettuce

3 Granny Smith apples,
    peeled and cored

2 stalks celery

¼" ginger, peeled

2 cups purified water

1. Combine romaine, apples, celery, ginger, and 1 cup of water in a blender and blend until thoroughly combined.
2. Add remaining 1 cup of water as needed while blending until desired consistency is achieved.

	Calories	Fat	Protein	Sodium	Fiber	Carbohydrates
PER 1 CUP SERVING	64	0g	1g	19mg	2g	17g

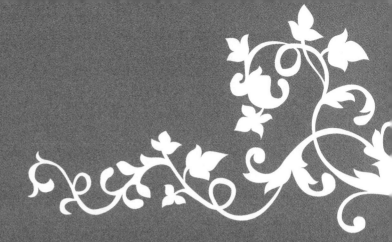

CHAPTER 4
Juices

Watermelon, cranberries, carrots, cucumbers, and more—there are plenty of tasty fruit and vegetable juices to choose from in this section. With ingredient combinations to help curb pregnancy cravings and others to help deal with morning sickness, there's a benefit to each of these delicious drinks. Now it's just a matter of choosing which one to whip up!

Kale Apple

Good for your baby's nervous system

Kale, a member of the cabbage family, is packed with folate, which is vital to forming your baby's brain and nervous system. Kale, a less commonly consumed cruciferous vegetable, is a good source of vitamins A and C, folic acid, iron, and calcium. In other words, it's perfect for building your baby's bones.

YIELDS: ¾ CUP

2 Granny Smith apples, cored
1 kale leaf

Juice apples and kale. Stir.

	Calories	Fat	Protein	Sodium	Fiber	Carbohydrates
PER ¾ CUP SERVING	112	0.62g	0.94g	14mg	4.3g	25g

Carrot Banana

This juice is highly nutritious and provides potassium, vitamin A, and vitamin C for both you and your baby-to-be. Carrots also provide vitamin A, making this juice so important for the development of your baby's eyes, teeth, and bones. In addition, the fiber content of the carrots in this recipe will help keep your digestive system balanced during your pregnancy!

YIELDS: 1 CUP

3 carrots

1 banana

Juice carrots. Add carrot juice and banana to blender and blend well.

	Calories	Fat	Protein	Sodium	Fiber	Carbohydrates
PER 1 CUP SERVING	274	0.49g	4.6g	118mg	13g	64g

AVOID DISCOLORED BANANAS

Once bananas are peeled and exposed to the air they begin to turn brown. If you want to peel your banana ahead of time, soak it in acidulated water (water with a few drops of lemon juice) to keep it from turning brown.

Popeye's Rescue

This juice is high in magnesium, a natural muscle relaxant, which will keep you feeling relaxed. In addition, spinach is very rich in iron and folic acid. It is a great source of vitamins A, C, and B$_6$, which not only support your baby's tissue and brain growth, but may also help with your morning sickness.

YIELDS: 1 CUP

1 cup spinach leaves
1 cucumber, peeled
2 carrots, peeled

Juice spinach, cucumber, and carrots. Stir.

	Calories	Fat	Protein	Sodium	Fiber	Carbohydrates
PER 1 CUP SERVING	125	0.13g	3.9g	106mg	7.6g	39g

Mango Kiwifruit

Good for fighting infections during pregnancy

The fear of getting sick or having fewer treatment options during pregnancy can be put to rest with this immune booster. Mangos are high in vitamins A and C, beta-carotene, niacin, fiber, and potassium, all of which help fight infection and toxins. In addition, kiwifruit contain more vitamin C than oranges, and they're also high in antioxidants, which allow you to prevent those common colds or, if you do get sick, recover from them more quickly.

YIELDS: 1 CUP

2 mangos, pitted
3 kiwifruit, peeled

Juice mango and kiwi. Stir well before serving.

	Calories	Fat	Protein	Sodium	Fiber	Carbohydrates
PER 1 CUP SERVING	273	3.1g	4.4g	11 mg	11g	95g

Pineapple Greets Papaya

Good for your digestive system

If you experience a change in your digestive tract during pregnancy, this juice contains the best nutrients for your tummy health. Bromelain, a digestive enzyme found in pineapple, can help restore normal digestion, and papaya is a good source of vitamins A and C, which help remove waste products that can slow digestion.

1 cup pineapple

½ orange

1 papaya, seeded

Juice pineapple, orange, and papaya. Stir well.

	Calories	Fat	Protein	Sodium	Fiber	Carbohydrates
PER 1½ CUP SERVING	134	0.42g	3.7mg	2.2g	5g	35g

Cabbage Juice

Cabbage is high in vitamins C and K, fiber, and detoxifying sulfur compounds, which can assist in fighting off several germs found in common public places, like offices, restrooms, and schools. This juice will keep you and your baby-to-be healthy.

1 cup chopped cabbage
2 carrots, peeled
2 apples, cored

Juice cabbage, carrots, and apples. Stir.

	Calories	Fat	Protein	Sodium	Fiber	Carbohydrates
PER 1¼ CUP SERVING	180	0.38g	3.3g	95mg	11g	54g

Cranberry Apple

Good for fighting infections during pregnancy

Pregnancy increases your risk for urinary infections, and incorporating the cranberry juice found in this recipe into your diet will help prevent bacteria from sticking to your bladder. Cranberries are very high in vitamin C. They're only in season for a few months, but fresh berries purchased in November and December can be frozen and used throughout the year.

YIELDS: 1 CUP

1¼ cups cranberries
2 red apples, cored

Juice cranberries and apples. Stir.

	Calories	Fat	Protein	Sodium	Fiber	Carbohydrates
PER 1 CUP SERVING	76	0.31g	1g	1.7mg	3.6g	27g

Watermelon Straight Up

Helps boost energy levels

Watermelon is very high in electrolytes, so this sweet treat is a glass of energy when you need it most during your pregnancy. Electrolytes help regulate your body's fluids, which helps you maintain a healthy pH balance and supports an optimal level of body function. With this juice, your energy levels will also be more than efficient.

YIELDS: 1 CUP

1 cup watermelon, rind removed
1 lime, peeled

Juice watermelon and lime. Stir.

	Calories	Fat	Protein	Sodium	Fiber	Carbohydrates
PER 1 CUP SERVING	65	0.32g	2.2g	2.8mg	2g	20

Immune Booster

Good for fighting infections during pregnancy

If you're exercising during pregnancy, this is the perfect juice to help strengthen those recovering muscles. The turnips, carrots, and watercress found in this recipe are good sources of vitamin C, which helps to fight off infections. Turnip is a root vegetable whose flavor varies from sweet to woody. It will keep for a long time in the refrigerator.

YIELDS: 1¼ CUP

1 apple, cored
1 turnip
2 carrots, peeled
½ cup watercress

Juice apple, turnip, carrots, and watercress. Stir.

	Calories	Fat	Protein	Sodium	Fiber	Carbohydrates
PER 1¼ CUP SERVING	177	0.34g	3.8g	200mg	11g	50g

Sinus Cleanser

Radishes are roots in the mustard family that are available year round. Their flavor is somewhat mild but has a peppery finish. The spiciness of the radish should help clear your sinus passages without medication, which many providers recommend you stay away from throughout pregnancy. And, while some spicy foods may not agree with your sensitive stomach during pregnancy, radishes may curb nausea in the first trimester by reducing the acid in your stomach.

2 tomatoes

4 radishes

Juice tomatoes and radishes. Stir.

	Calories	Fat	Protein	Sodium	Fiber	Carbohydrates
PER ¾ CUP SERVING	50	0.31g	2.7g	41mg	3g	9g

Cranberry Orange

Good for fighting infections during pregnancy

This juice will be most important for warding off any potential infections and may even prevent the need for any medications during your pregnancy. Fresh cranberries and oranges are very high in vitamin C, which will protect your body. In addition, cranberries have compounds called proanthocyanidins that will keep harmful bacteria from sticking to your bladder.

YIELDS: ½ CUP

2 cups cranberries

1 orange, peeled

Juice cranberries and orange.

	Calories	Fat	Protein	Sodium	Fiber	Carbohydrates
PER ½ CUP SERVING	152	0.56g	2.1g	3.8mg	12g	44g

Strawberry Papaya

Good for fighting infections during pregnancy

The last thing you want is for your immune system not to be in its best shape during your pregnancy. Nothing's worse than being sick if you're already not feeling your best! Fortunately, the strawberries and papayas found in this recipe are both known to help fight infections due to their high vitamin C content. In addition, the banana provides vitamin B$_6$ for extra immune-system support.

YIELDS: ½ CUP

1 cup strawberries, hulls intact
1 papaya, seeded and peeled
1 banana, peeled

Juice berries and papaya separately. Blend juices in a blender.
Add banana and blend until smooth.

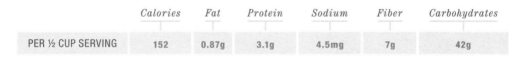

	Calories	Fat	Protein	Sodium	Fiber	Carbohydrates
PER ½ CUP SERVING	152	0.87g	3.1g	4.5mg	7g	42g

White Grape and Lime

Look for fresh green grapes that have a pale color for this refreshing drink. The abundance of minerals found in grapes helps to detoxify the liver and strengthens your digestive system to help ensure you're absorbing as many nutrients as you can during your pregnancy.

YIELDS: 1 CUP

1½ cups green seedless grapes
2 limes, peeled

Juice grapes and limes.

	Calories	Fat	Protein	Sodium	Fiber	Carbohydrates
PER 1 CUP SERVING	70	0.45g	1.8g	3.6mg	4.5g	38g

Tropical Cucumber

Good for healthy skin and hair

It's important to feel your best both inside and out, especially while you're pregnant, and the cucumber in this delicious drink provides a multitude of skin benefits. Cucumber contains silica, a trace mineral that helps provide strength to the connective tissues of the skin, which can help with swelling of the eyes and water retention. Cucumbers are also high in vitamins A and C and folic acid.

YIELDS: 2 CUPS

1 cup pineapple, peeled and cut into chunks
1 mango, pitted
1 cucumber, peeled
½ lemon, rind intact

Juice pineapple first, then mango and cucumber. Cut lemon into thin slices and juice last. Stir well before serving.

	Calories	Fat	Protein	Sodium	Fiber	Carbohydrates
PER 2 CUP SERVING	163	0.53g	3.9g	8.8mg	6.9g	52g

Apple Grape

Some studies have shown that apple consumption during pregnancy reduces risk for childhood wheezing and asthma. Note: Apple seeds may not be juiced because they contain cyanide, which is poisonous. Make sure you remove the seeds from the apple before placing it through the juicer.

YIELDS: 1 CUP

2 red Gala apples, cored
1 cup green seedless grapes

Juice apples first, then juice grapes. Stir well before serving.

	Calories	Fat	Protein	Sodium	Fiber	Carbohydrates
PER 1 CUP SERVING	126	0.58g	0.91g	3.1mg	3.4g	53g

Apple Lemonade

While apples are key players in maintaining a healthy digestive system during your pregnancy, pesticides should not be invited to the game. Unfortunately, the placement of apples on the "Dirty Dozen" list put out yearly by the Environmental Working Group (EWG) makes it especially important to purchase organic apples, whose skins won't have come into contact with anything dangerous.

2 red Gala apples, cored
2 Granny Smith apples, cored
¼ lemon, rind intact

Juice apples first. Cut lemon into thin slices and then juice them. Stir.

	Calories	Fat	Protein	Sodium	Fiber	Carbohydrates
PER 1 CUP SERVING	135	0.65g	0.27g	3.3mg	6.3g	38g

Apple Celery

Good for healthy skin and hair

Celery is rich in silica that can balance the tone and firmness of your skin during pregnancy. It also helps your skin retain water and stay hydrated, which will keep you glowing throughout your pregnancy. Let's drink to good health—and beautiful skin!

1 Granny Smith apple, cored
2 stalks celery

Juice apples and celery. Stir well.

	Calories	Fat	Protein	Sodium	Fiber	Carbohydrates
PER 1¼ CUP SERVING	47	0.36g	1g	82mg	3.3g	12g

Apple Banana

Good for healthy skin and hair

This juice will make you feel you're taking care of your inner and outer beauty, from skin and hair to supporting your baby's lungs and overall growth. The apples used in this recipe are packed with vitamins and minerals, including vitamins C and A, folate, potassium, and iron that play an important role in the development of healthy glowing skin.

YIELDS: 1 CUP

3 Granny Smith apples, cored
1 lemon, peeled
1 banana, peeled

Juice apples and lemon. Add banana and blend in a blender until smooth.

	Calories	Fat	Protein	Sodium	Fiber	Carbohydrates
PER 1 CUP SERVING	190	0.9g	1.4g	3.9mg	8.1g	51g

Berry Cherry

Good news! Cherries are an excellent source of vitamin C, which plays a role in the production of collagen. Collagen plays a part in your skin's ability to rebound after stretching, which is great because, as you've noticed, your body's shape is rapidly changing throughout your pregnancy.

YIELDS: 1 CUP

1 cup cherries, pitted
1½ cups strawberries
1 pint raspberries

Juice cherries, strawberries, and raspberries.

	Calories	Fat	Protein	Sodium	Fiber	Carbohydrates
PER 1 CUP SERVING	279	2.9g	6.8g	9.4mg	24g	67g

Kale Apple Spinach

This juice contains folate, which helps prevent neurological birth defects in your baby. The Centers for Disease Control and Prevention reports that women who take the recommended daily dose of folic acid starting at least one month before they conceive and during the first trimester reduce their baby's risk of neural tube defects by 50–70 percent. Folate is also responsible for the genetic map of your baby. The recommendation from experts is to have 400mcg of folic acid per day.

YIELDS: 1¼ CUPS

2 red apples, cored
2 carrots, peeled
4 large kale leaves
1 cup spinach

Juice apples, carrots, kale, and spinach. Stir.

	Calories	Fat	Protein	Sodium	Fiber	Carbohydrates
PER 1¼ CUP SERVING	295	2.9g	16g	400mg	18g	57g

Ginger Carrot Beet

All beets are full of folic acid, vitamin C, and potassium, but red beets also provide vitamins A and C, calcium, iron, and fiber. Thanks to the humble beet, this delicious juice will assist in the development of your baby's heart, lungs, kidneys, eyes, and bones, and his circulatory, respiratory, and central nervous systems.

YIELDS: 1 CUP

4 carrots, peeled
¼" slice gingerroot
1 beet, rinsed

Juice carrots, ginger, and beet. Stir.

	Calories	Fat	Protein	Sodium	Fiber	Carbohydrates
PER 1 CUP SERVING	231	0.27g	5.8g	222mg	15g	60g

Sunshine in a Glass

This juice contains vitamin C that boosts both your and your baby's immune systems. The antioxidants that come from vitamin C are so tough that it's like hiring bodyguards to protect your and your baby's immune system. And, when it comes to protecting your baby-to-be, a little hired muscle can't hurt, right?

2 red Gala apples, cored
1½ cups strawberries, hulls intact
¼ lime, rind intact

Cut apples into thin slices. Juice apples first and then strawberries.
Cut lime into thin slices and juice. Stir well.

	Calories	Fat	Protein	Sodium	Fiber	Carbohydrates
PER 1½ CUP SERVING	143	1.1g	2.4g	3.9mg	7.5g	52g

Cherry Cucumber

Sleep patterns can change dramatically throughout your pregnancy due to hormonal changes and discomfort. Thankfully, cherries contain melatonin, a hormone that helps control your sleep and wake cycles, and their addition in this delicious juice will keep you calm and help you sleep. Enjoy it while you can!

YIELDS: 1½ CUPS

1 cucumber, peeled
2 cups red sweet cherries, pitted
2 stalks celery, leaves intact

Juice cucumber, cherries, and celery. Stir.

	Calories	Fat	Protein	Sodium	Fiber	Carbohydrates
PER 1½ CUP SERVING	221	0.81g	5.1g	85mg	9.1g	53g

Papaya Delight

The ingredients in this delicious juice are packed full of magnesium, which helps build and repair your tissues throughout pregnancy. In fact, a severe magnesium deficiency can lead to preeclampsia, high blood pressure during pregnancy, that affects 5 percent of all pregnant women and may lead to poor fetal growth or preterm labor. So, cheers to this Papaya Delight and to a healthy baby!

YIELDS: 1½ CUPS

1 cup pineapple, peeled
7 large strawberries, hulls intact
½ papaya, seeds removed

Juice pineapple, strawberries, and papaya.

	Calories	Fat	Protein	Sodium	Fiber	Carbohydrates
PER 1½ CUP SERVING	166	0.91g	4.3g	5.7mg	6.9g	36g

Peach Strawberry

Peaches can enrich your pregnancy in multiple ways, because they are full of folic acid; vitamins A, C, and E; and potassium. This juice will help prevent birth defects, support your baby's growth, boost your immune system, improve your skin, and help you stay hydrated.

YIELDS: 1¼ CUPS

1 large peach, pitted
7 large strawberries, hulls intact

Juice peach and then strawberries. Stir.

	Calories	Fat	Protein	Sodium	Fiber	Carbohydrates
PER 1¼ CUP SERVING	124	1g	3.5g	2mg	7.1g	28g

Dilly of a Cucumber

Good for your baby's bones and development

The cucumbers used in this recipe are a great source of folate, which is particularly important during pregnancy as it can help reduce the risk of neural-tube defects in your baby. Cucumbers are also a good source of the antioxidant vitamins A and C, which assist in growth and healthy development.

YIELDS: 1¼ CUPS

½ large cucumber, peeled
1 stalk celery, leaves intact
2 sprigs fresh baby dill

Juice cucumber. Add celery and juice to combine. Stir well.
Garnish with fresh sprigs of dill.

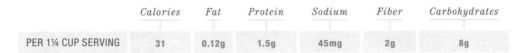

	Calories	Fat	Protein	Sodium	Fiber	Carbohydrates
PER 1¼ CUP SERVING	31	0.12g	1.5g	45mg	2g	8g

FRESH DILL

Dill is a tasty herb and a nice addition to this drink. However, dill does not juice through your juicer, so the best thing to do is serve your cucumber drink with a fresh sprig of it. If you want more dill flavor, add chopped dill to the drink.

Carrot Apple Broccoli

Good for your baby's bones and development

The broccoli found in this juice will build your baby's bones and keep yours strong. Broccoli is a good source of vitamin C, but it also contains riboflavin, calcium, and iron. The vitamin C and calcium are key players when it comes to strengthening your bones and riboflavin promotes your baby's growth, vision, healthy skin, and bone and muscle development.

YIELDS: 1¼ CUPS

2 carrots, peeled

1 red delicious apple, cored

1 cup broccoli

Juice carrots, apple, and then broccoli. Stir.

	Calories	Fat	Protein	Sodium	Fiber	Carbohydrates
PER 1¼ CUP SERVING	157	0.44g	4.7g	109mg	10g	44g

Cherry and Blueberry

There are about sixteen varieties of blueberry. They have more antioxidants than any other fruit or vegetable, and they're also high in fiber, potassium, and vitamins A and C. All of these antioxidants and nutrients will help protect you and your baby from any foreign molecules that should not be hanging around. Therefore, you'll have a stronger immune system and a healthy digestive system, and will support your baby's growth.

YIELDS: 1¼ CUPS

1 cup sweet cherries, pitted

2 cups blueberries

Juice cherries and blueberries. Stir.

	Calories	Fat	Protein	Sodium	Fiber	Carbohydrates
PER 1¼ CUP SERVING	257	1.3g	4.4g	2.9mg	8.8g	61g

Lettuce Patch

Helps boost energy levels

As your iron needs increase during pregnancy, your energy levels can suffer. However, the parsnip power in this juice can provide you with iron and vitamin C in order to absorb that iron. If you don't absorb iron, your body won't be able to efficiently produce hemoglobin that carries oxygen to your cells, which can lead to fatigue or anemia. Fortunately, the vitamin C and iron combination found in this recipe will increase your energy levels and keep you feeling great!

YIELDS: 1½ CUPS

1 cup romaine lettuce

1 parsnip

½ cup spinach

1 carrot, peeled

Juice ingredients in order listed. Stir well before serving.

	Calories	Fat	Protein	Sodium	Fiber	Carbohydrates
PER 1½ CUP SERVING	165	0.65g	3.6g	69mg	11g	39g

PARSNIPS

Parsnips came to America in the early seventeenth century, but their popularity didn't take off immediately. They are a white root vegetable that is available year round. They contain vitamin C and iron and will last for up to two weeks in your fridge if kept in a plastic bag.

Savoy and Broccoli

Good for strengthening your immune system

The ingredients in this juice are packed full of vitamin C, which means that this juice can protect your and your baby's immune systems throughout your pregnancy. This juice is perfect when you're not feeling up for a big bowl of greens.

YIELDS: ¾ CUP

1 cup broccoli

3 leaves red lettuce

¼ head Savoy cabbage

Juice ingredients in order listed. Stir well before serving.

	Calories	Fat	Protein	Sodium	Fiber	Carbohydrates
PER ¾ CUP SERVING	77	0.55g	6.2g	82mg	7.5g	12g

Carrot Kale

The ginger found in this recipe is said to ease the symptoms of morning sickness that can be common in the beginning of your pregnancy. In addition, the calcium and vitamins A and C found in the carrots, apples, and kale will also protect your and your baby's bone health. What's better than that?

YIELDS: 1 CUP

2 carrots, peeled
¼" slice gingerroot
1 red apple, cored
2 leaves kale
¼ cup parsley

Juice carrots, ginger, and apple. Juice kale and parsley. Stir together.

	Calories	Fat	Protein	Sodium	Fiber	Carbohydrates
PER 1 CUP SERVING	162	0.73g	3.7g	111mg	8.4g	40g

Snap Pea Smoothie

This juice is packed with vitamins A, K, and C, and manganese, which makes it perfect for pregnancy! The vitamins all play a key role in the development of your baby from her bones to her heart, and manganese helps form bone and cartilage, which will support your baby's bones. This juice also provides fiber from snap peas that will support a healthy digestive system and prevent hemorrhoids, which can be more common in pregnancy. Drink up!

YIELDS: ¾ CUP

1 cup snap peas
2 carrots, peeled
2 stalks celery

Juice snap peas, carrots, and celery. Stir.

	Calories	Fat	Protein	Sodium	Fiber	Carbohydrates
PER ¾ CUP SERVING	142	0.35g	5.2g	166mg	11g	39g

Salad in a Glass

Good for your baby's bones and development

When you're not in the mood for a salad, the broccoli and carrots in this juice can provide you and your baby with adequate nutrition and strengthen your baby's bones. You can vary this recipe by switching the lettuce to romaine lettuce or red leaf lettuce.

YIELDS: 1 CUP

1 cup broccoli
3 leaves butterhead lettuce
1 carrot
2 red radishes
1 green onion

Juice ingredients in order listed. Stir. Garnish glass with green onion tops.

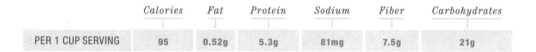

	Calories	Fat	Protein	Sodium	Fiber	Carbohydrates
PER 1 CUP SERVING	95	0.52g	5.3g	81mg	7.5g	21g

BUTTERHEAD LETTUCE

Butterhead lettuce is small and round. Its leaves have a soft buttery texture, and the flavor is sweet. Gentle washing is required for this type of lettuce because it is delicate.

Pineapple Plum Punch

The pineapple and plums in this juice are packed with magnesium, which can help strengthen your bones. However, magnesium is often used to treat preeclampsia or preterm labor during pregnancy, so you should talk to your doctor before consuming this juice.

YIELDS: 1½ CUPS

2 black plums
1 cup pineapple

Juice plums and pineapple. Stir well before serving.

	Calories	Fat	Protein	Sodium	Fiber	Carbohydrates
PER 1½ CUP SERVING	136	0.62g	2.9g	1.6mg	2.9g	35g

HOW TO CHOOSE A PINEAPPLE

Choose a pineapple that is a bit soft to the touch. It should not show signs of green. The leaves should be green with no brown spots. If a pineapple is overripe it will have soft areas on the skin. If you purchase a pineapple that isn't ripe you may keep it at room temperature for a few days. If you cannot find fresh pineapple, choose a canned variety that's been packed in its own juice.

Strawberry Patch

Good for strengthening your immune system

Strawberries are a great source of vitamin C, iron, and potassium, which makes them perfect for boosting your immune system. If you cannot get fresh berries, feel free to substitute organic frozen strawberries for this juice.

YIELDS: 1 CUP

1 apple, cored
1 cup strawberries, hulls intact

Juice apple and then strawberries. Stir well before serving.

	Calories	Fat	Protein	Sodium	Fiber	Carbohydrates
PER 1 CUP SERVING	81	0.64g	1.5g	2.1mg	4.3g	30g

Purple Cow

Spinach, turnip greens, and broccoli are all rich in calcium, vitamin C, and iron. These nutrients are helpful during pregnancy to prevent anemia and in building your baby's bones. The protein from milk and fiber from berries will also help sustain your energy levels by balancing your blood sugars.

YIELDS: 1½ CUPS

1 cup blueberries
1 pint blackberries
½ cup skim milk

Juice berries. Stir in milk.

	Calories	Fat	Protein	Sodium	Fiber	Carbohydrates
PER 1½ CUP SERVING	250	2g	8.5g	68mg	17g	55g

Strawberry Pineapple Grape

Good for strengthening your immune system

This juice is an incredibly delicious way to build your immune system! The grapes, pineapple, and strawberries used here contain a bundle of vitamin C that creates the antioxidants that protect your tissues from damage. Vitamin C is also essential for tissue repair, wound healing, bone growth and repair, and healthy skin.

YIELDS: 1½ CUPS

1 cup pineapple

1 cup red grapes

1 cup strawberries, hulls intact

Juice pineapple, grapes, and strawberries. Stir before serving.

	Calories	Fat	Protein	Sodium	Fiber	Carbohydrates
PER 1½ CUP SERVING	184	0.98g	4g	4.9mg	5.5g	66g

Cantaloupe Straight Up

One cup of cantaloupe contains almost your daily requirement for antioxidants. Since anti-oxidants are the bodyguards of your system, this juice will protect your body from any free radicals wanting to cause damage. Cantaloupe is also a good source of potassium, vitamin B_6, dietary fiber, and niacin (vitamin B_3). Potassium will support your hydration status throughout your pregnancy and B_6 and fiber will help you sustain healthy energy levels. In addition, niacin helps turn food into energy and assists with the development of your baby.

YIELDS: 1 CUP

½ cantaloupe, seeds and rind removed

Juice cantaloupe.

	Calories	Fat	Protein	Sodium	Fiber	Carbohydrates
PER 1 CUP SERVING	121	0.79g	3.6g	57mg	3.6g	14g

Watermelon Lime Cherry

Watermelon can help alleviate heartburn and can reduce uncomfortable swelling during your pregnancy. How? Well, its high potassium levels and high water content allows it to flush what may be causing your heartburn or swelling out of your system, while keeping you hydrated at the same time. Watermelon is also full of vitamins A, C, and B$_6$, as well as potassium and magnesium, which are important for your baby's immune and nervous systems.

YIELDS: 1 CUP

1 cup watermelon, rind removed
1 cup cherries, pitted
½ lime

Juice watermelon, cherries, and lime. Stir.

	Calories	Fat	Protein	Sodium	Fiber	Carbohydrates
PER 1 CUP SERVING	134	0.77g	3.4g	6.9mg	4.1g	35g

Nightcap Smoothie

This juice is perfect for when you notice your sleeping patterns changing throughout your pregnancy. Lettuce has a sedative effect that helps promote sleep and the high amounts of calcium found in this ingredient also helps your muscles relax, allowing you to sleep better.

YIELDS: 1 CUP

2 carrots, peeled
2 stalks celery
2 leaves romaine lettuce

Juice carrots, celery, and lettuce. Stir.

	Calories	Fat	Protein	Sodium	Fiber	Carbohydrates
PER 1 CUP SERVING	110	0.26g	3.1g	160mg	8.3g	29g

Go to Sleep Smoothie

Since your body is trying to accommodate a new person, you might feel more tired during your pregnancy and a good night's sleep will help you stay feeling your best. If you're tired, your body is going to have to put the energy it has available to support your energy levels and less will be available for your baby. Fortunately, the parsley found in this recipe is a good source of calcium and magnesium, both of which are known to promote healthy sleep patterns.

YIELDS: 1 CUP

4 carrots, peeled
2 stalks celery
2 leaves romaine lettuce
⅛ cup parsley

Juice carrots, celery, and romaine. Stir. Garnish with parsley.

	Calories	Fat	Protein	Sodium	Fiber	Carbohydrates
PER 1 CUP SERVING	207	0.26g	5.1g	242mg	14g	55g

Carrot and Cauliflower

Celery is rich in vitamin C, potassium, and folic acid. Vitamin C is great for tissue repair and bone growth and repair during pregnancy and potassium will help your body stay hydrated so it can work as efficiently as possible to support the optimal growth and health of your baby-to-be. In addition, the folic acid found here in its naturally occurring state, is essential for the functioning of DNA and cell growth of your baby. Talk about an easy way to get some healthy benefits!

YIELDS: 1¼ CUPS

4 leaves romaine lettuce
3 carrots, peeled
½ cup cauliflower
½ lemon, peeled

Juice ingredients in order listed. Stir.

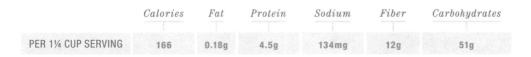

	Calories	Fat	Protein	Sodium	Fiber	Carbohydrates
PER 1¼ CUP SERVING	166	0.18g	4.5g	134mg	12g	51g

Ultimate "C" Energizer

Helps boost energy levels

During pregnancy, you will have almost 50 percent more blood in your system to meet the demands of your growing uterus and protect you and your baby from harm when you lie down or stand up. This means that the amount of iron in your body needs increase to manage the additional red blood cells and to prevent anemia due to the increase in plasma. Fortunately, this citrus delight is full of the mighty vitamin C, which helps your body better absorb iron. And the more iron you can absorb, the more energy you'll have in stock.

YIELDS: 1½ CUPS

2 oranges, peeled
½ pink grapefruit, peeled
½ lemon, peeled

Juice oranges and grapefruit. Juice lemon. Stir.

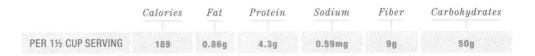

	Calories	*Fat*	*Protein*	*Sodium*	*Fiber*	*Carbohydrates*
PER 1½ CUP SERVING	189	0.86g	4.3g	0.59mg	9g	50g

Wake Up Watercress Smoothie

Helps boost energy levels

Watercress is a member of the mustard family and due to its iron content, is often recommended as a vegetable that can help pregnant women who are anemic or at risk for developing anemia during pregnancy. You will need this extra iron for your growing baby and placenta, especially in the second and third trimesters, when the amount of blood in your body increases to protect your baby.

YIELDS: ¾ CUP

1 apple, cored
1 cup spinach leaves
1 handful watercress

Juice apple, spinach, and watercress. Stir.

	Calories	*Fat*	*Protein*	*Sodium*	*Fiber*	*Carbohydrates*
PER ¾ CUP SERVING	39	0.27g	0.91g	25mg	1.9g	13g

Orange Lemonade Lift-Off

Helps boost energy levels

This citrusy juice is packed with vitamin C, which means you'll actually have the energy to go to the supermarket or the gym instead of just wanting to go right to bed! Sleep is important, but when you feel as good as this juice will make you feel, don't waste the energy!

YIELDS: ¾ CUP

3 oranges, peeled
1 lemon, peeled

Juice oranges and lemon. Stir.

	Calories	Fat	Protein	Sodium	Fiber	Carbohydrates
PER ¾ CUP SERVING	211	1.1g	4.8g	1.2mg	10g	56g

Apple Banana High

Let's face it, pregnancy can be exhausting. Fortunately, the vitamin C found in the lemon and banana used in this recipe helps your body absorb all the iron in this drink that comes from the blackberries. Efficient iron absorption is essential for carrying oxygen to your cells to ensure your baby is receiving the nutrients you're providing, especially during pregnancy.

YIELDS: 1¼ CUPS

2 Granny Smith apples
1 pint blackberries
1 lemon
1 banana

Juice apples, blackberries, and lemon. Add banana to juice and stir well before serving.

	Calories	Fat	Protein	Sodium	Fiber	Carbohydrates
PER 1¼ CUP SERVING	287	2.2g	4.8g	8.2mg	25g	80g

Razzle Dazzle Berry

Both raspberries and strawberries are rich in vitamin C, which provides an abundance of antioxidants to protect you and your baby from free radicals that are trying to cause damage. This keeps both you and your baby-to-be's immune systems strong and helps you reach your optimal health during pregnancy. Try this mix of strawberries and raspberries for a really rich drink that is easy to make.

YIELDS: 1 CUP

2 cups strawberries, hulls intact
1 pint raspberries

Juice berries. Stir before serving.

	Calories	Fat	Protein	Sodium	Fiber	Carbohydrates
PER 1 CUP SERVING	222	2.3g	5.9g	5.9mg	21g	63g

Pineapple Tangerine

Helps boost energy levels

Let's face it, the increased stress on your body over the next nine months may put you into a state of fatigue. Fortunately, the pineapples and tangerines used in this delicious juice are both good sources of iron and vitamin C, which can improve your stamina and circulation to increase your energy levels.

YIELDS: 1 CUP

1 cup pineapple, peeled
1 tangerine, peeled

Juice pineapple and tangerine. Stir.

	Calories	Fat	Protein	Sodium	Fiber	Carbohydrates
PER 1 CUP SERVING	127	0.0g	2.4g	3.5mg	3.3g	33g

Pineapple Cucumber

Pineapples and cucumbers are both good for treating edema, the accumulation of fluid beneath the skin. Pineapples stimulate the kidneys to remove excess water from the body and the high water content in cucumbers will help you avoid dehydration, another common way to develop edema.

YIELDS: 1 CUP

1 English cucumber, peeled
1 cup pineapple, peeled

Juice cucumber and pineapple. Stir. Garnish with cube of pineapple on a stick.

	Calories	Fat	Protein	Sodium	Fiber	Carbohydrates
PER 1 CUP SERVING	99	0.17g	2.6g	5.6mg	2.6g	32g

Cauliflower Broccoli

Helps boost energy levels

B vitamins are well known to increase your energy levels, which are hard to sustain during pregnancy. Vitamin B is the key to this energy-boosting juice, and the magnesium in the cauliflower and beet greens will also keep you on your feet . . . and off the couch!

1 cup cauliflower
4 spears broccoli
2 beet greens

Juice cauliflower, broccoli, and beet greens separately. Stir together.

	Calories	Fat	Protein	Sodium	Fiber	Carbohydrates
PER 1 CUP SERVING	78	0.56g	6.7g	213mg	9g	10g

Grapefruit Star

If you've ever been down with the flu while pregnant, you know how hard it is to be sick without running to the pharmacy and grabbing the first over-the-counter cold and flu remedy that you can find. The good news is that the vitamin C found in this recipe is just the thing to get you through a bout of the common cold or flu without medication. This juice may also keep you from catching a cold in the first place . . . and prevention is better than a cure anyway!

YIELDS: 1 CUP

½ pink grapefruit, rind removed
½ white grapefruit, rind removed

Juice grapefruits. Stir.

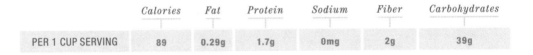

	Calories	Fat	Protein	Sodium	Fiber	Carbohydrates
PER 1 CUP SERVING	89	0.29g	1.7g	0mg	2g	39g

Broccoli and Kale

Good for strengthening your immune system

You know that citrus fruits contain vitamin C, but you may not have heard that broccoli and kale are particularly good sources of this super vitamin as well. In addition to protecting you and your baby from free radicals that may cause harm, vitamin C repairs tissues, support the growth of your baby's bones, helps your body fight infections, and promotes healthy skin throughout your pregnancy. Sounds like a super vitamin!

YIELDS: 1 CUP

2 leaves kale
1 beet top and greens
1 fistful spinach
½ cup broccoli florets

Juice ingredients in order listed. Stir.

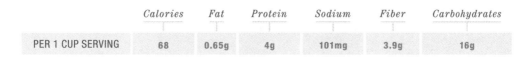

	Calories	Fat	Protein	Sodium	Fiber	Carbohydrates
PER 1 CUP SERVING	68	0.65g	4g	101mg	3.9g	16g

Spinach Apple

Spinach is rich in iron and vitamins A, C, and E, all of which help protect your baby from infection and your cells from damage. Spinach is also good for calcium absorption and it helps cleanse the intestinal tract and relieve constipation, an unfortunate pregnancy side effect. It also has a higher protein content than other leafy greens.

1 cup spinach leaves, washed and dried
1 red apple
¼ lemon, rind intact
1 stalk celery

Juice spinach, apple, lemon, and celery. Stir.

	Calories	Fat	Protein	Sodium	Fiber	Carbohydrates
PER ¾ CUP SERVING	84	0.61g	1.7g	67mg	5.5g	16g

Butternut Delight

Good for your baby's bones and development

This juice is not only important for your baby's development, but also for you. Butternut squash is a great source of vitamin A, which is crucial during pregnancy and helps with your baby's bone growth, eye development, skin health, and infection resistance.

2 Gala apples, cored
½ butternut squash, peeled and cut into pieces
1 teaspoon pumpkin pie spice

Juice apples and squash. Stir in pumpkin pie spice.

	Calories	Fat	Protein	Sodium	Fiber	Carbohydrates
PER 1 CUP SERVING	159	0.42g	2.8g	12 mg	6.9g	57g

Citrus Cucumber

Good for your digestive system

The cucumbers used in this recipe are 90 percent water. Their high water content keeps the inside of the cucumber much cooler than the surrounding atmosphere and makes it a good diuretic, which works to flush toxins from your body that may cause cramping or bloating in your digestion system during pregnancy. The high water content in cucumbers will also keep you hydrated throughout your pregnancy, which is required to assist every action needed for developing a healthy baby.

YIELDS: 1½ CUPS

1 pink grapefruit, peeled
1 orange, peeled
¼" slice ginger
1 cucumber, peeled

Juice grapefruit, orange, ginger, and cucumber. Stir.

	Calories	Fat	Protein	Sodium	Fiber	Carbohydrates
PER 1½ CUP SERVING	202	0.73g	4.7g	5.1mg	7.6g	42g

Italian Carrot

Good for your digestive system

Your intestines may suffer from all that is happening during pregnancy, as in their new arrangement, they are pushed up and toward the sides as the uterus grows. The parsley juice used in this recipe is rich in beta-carotene and vitamins A and C, which are good for repairing any damage that has been done to your digestive system. In addition, carrots promote the healing of the intestine membranes.

YIELDS: 1 CUP

4 carrots, peeled
1 stalk celery
¼ cup Italian parsley

Juice carrots, celery, and parsley. Stir.

	Calories	Fat	Protein	Sodium	Fiber	Carbohydrates
PER 1 CUP SERVING	200	0.11g	4.5g	204mg	13g	53g

Ginger Carrot Apple

Good for morning sickness

The ginger used in this recipe contains compounds called ginerols, which act like anti-nausea medications and help block serotonin receptors in the stomach. Chances are, a drink that helps alleviate morning sickness will come in handy at some point during your pregnancy, probably within the first trimester when most women suffer from nausea and stomach pain.

YIELDS: ½ CUP

2 apples, cored

1 carrot, peeled

¼" slice ginger

Juice apples, carrot, and ginger. Stir.

	Calories	Fat	Protein	Sodium	Fiber	Carbohydrates
PER ½ CUP SERVING	119	0.36g	1.2g	41mg	5.7g	37g

Rise and Shine

Good for your digestive system

Heartburn and indigestion may seem to pop up out of nowhere during pregnancy, due to an increase in sensitivity to spicy or common irritating foods or acids that are backed up into the esophagus because your uterus is enlarging and displacing the stomach. Fortunately, the pineapple used in this juice can help you feel better fast by providing bromelain, an enzyme that helps assist protein digestion and acid reflux.

YIELDS: 1½ CUPS

1 cup pineapple
1 peach, pitted
1 mango, pitted
1 banana

Juice pineapple, peach, and mango. Add banana to juice and mix well before serving.

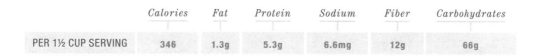

	Calories	Fat	Protein	Sodium	Fiber	Carbohydrates
PER 1½ CUP SERVING	346	1.3g	5.3g	6.6mg	12g	66g

Apricot Apple

Good for your digestive system

Apples provide an excellent source of both soluble and insoluble fiber, so they're great for helping you resolve constipation issues during pregnancy. After juicing the fruits, consider blending them with 1 cup of plain yogurt. Yogurt is very good for the stomach because it contains "good bacteria" that aids digestion.

YIELDS: 1 CUP

4 apricots, pitted
2 Gala apples, peeled

Juice apricots and apples. Stir.

	Calories	Fat	Protein	Sodium	Fiber	Carbohydrates
PER 1 CUP SERVING	107	0.56g	1.6g	1.1mg	3.4g	27g

Pear Apple

Good for your digestive system

The common occurrence of constipation during pregnancy may not be pleasant. However, the pectin in pears is a diuretic and so pears have a mild laxative effect. Drinking pear juice regularly helps regulate bowel movements. The Bartlett is known for being one of the most juicy pears, which is why it was selected for this recipe.

YIELDS: ¾ CUP

2 Bartlett pears
2 red delicious apples
¼ lemon, peeled

Juice pears, apples, and lemon. Stir.

	Calories	Fat	Protein	Sodium	Fiber	Carbohydrates
PER ¾ CUP SERVING	172	0.87g	2.6g	1.5mg	13g	51g

Apple Cucumber with a Twist

Good for your digestive system

This juice can be the perfect remedy for constipation. Apple skins have pectin, which helps remove harmful substances from the colon. Cucumbers contain an enzyme called erepsin that is useful in digesting protein. Enzymes that aid digestion are important during pregnancy to ensure that the nutrients from the foods you eat will be absorbed efficiently and delivered to your baby.

2 Granny Smith apples, cored

2 carrots, peeled

1 cucumber, peeled

1 lemon, peeled

1 stalk celery

Juice apples, carrots, cucumber, lemon, and celery. Stir.

	Calories	Fat	Protein	Sodium	Fiber	Carbohydrates
PER 1 CUP SERVING	263	1.6g	6.7g	226mg	17g	68g

Pear Pineapple

Good for your digestive system

The pears used in this recipe are a great source of fiber and pectin, both of which benefit your colon by aiding digestion, preventing constipation, and keeping things moving throughout your digestive system. In addition, pineapple has long been known for its ability to help with digestion due to the enzyme bromelain that aids in the digestion of proteins. Proteins are important during pregnancy for the growth of your fetus and play a huge part in increasing the blood supply for your baby.

YIELDS: 2 CUPS

½ pineapple, skin and core removed
2 Bartlett pears, cored
1 lemon, peeled

Juice pineapple, pears, and lemon. Stir.

	Calories	*Fat*	*Protein*	*Sodium*	*Fiber*	*Carbohydrates*
PER 2 CUP SERVING	372	0.94g	2g	7.7mg	18g	98g

Vegetable Seven

Tomatoes are high in the antioxidant lycopene, which can protect against cell damage caused by free radicals. You do not want any cell damage during pregnancy, because it can inhibit the optimal level of health of your baby. However, tomatoes are also acidic, which can cause heartburn or acid reflux during the second half of your pregnancy; if you're experiencing these symptoms, you may want to pass.

YIELDS: 1½ CUPS

2 Roma tomatoes
1 stalk celery, leaves intact
1 fistful parsley
2 carrots, peeled
1 green onion
1 cup cauliflower
2 cloves garlic

Blanch tomatoes by placing in boiling water for 30 seconds and then transferring to an ice bath. Juice ingredients in the order listed. Stir.

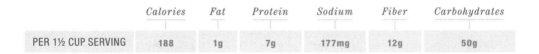

	Calories	Fat	Protein	Sodium	Fiber	Carbohydrates
PER 1½ CUP SERVING	188	1g	7g	177mg	12g	50g

THE BENEFITS OF LYCOPENE

Lycopene is a powerful antioxidant found in tomatoes. It has been shown to reduce the risk of prostate, ovarian, and cervical cancer and can protect your cells during pregnancy. To reap the benefits of lycopene, the tomatoes must be eaten cooked rather than raw.

Broccoli Apple Carrot

Broccoli is known for being a good source of calcium, but it is also packed with vitamin C, folate, and vitamin B_6, all of which work to support the bone health of you and your baby. B_6 is needed to make hydrochloric acid in the stomach, which helps your body absorb calcium and folate is important for lowering your baby's risk of developing a neurological birth defect. So drink up!

YIELDS: 1 CUP

4 spears broccoli
¼ cup Italian parsley
2 McIntosh apples, cored
¼ lemon

Juice broccoli, parsley, and apples. Juice lemon. Stir.

	Calories	Fat	Protein	Sodium	Fiber	Carbohydrates
PER 1 CUP SERVING	114	0.75g	3.7g	47mg	7.2g	27g

Garlic Delight

Helps boost energy levels

Good news! Garlic could potentially reduce fatigue during pregnancy. It can also protect you and your baby from harmful bacteria, fungi, and viruses. Garlic contains alliin, an amino acid that converts to allicin, a compound that has been shown to have antibiotic properties. It can also help improve blood circulation during pregnancy, which will reduce fatigue. So if you're craving Italian, you're in luck!

YIELDS: 1 CUP

3 Roma tomatoes

2 red apples

1 clove garlic

1 sprig Italian parsley

Juice tomatoes, apples, garlic, and parsley. Stir and garnish with parsley.

	Calories	Fat	Protein	Sodium	Fiber	Carbohydrates
PER 1 CUP SERVING	114	1.3g	2.4g	18mg	4.6g	44g

Carrot, Cucumber, and Beet

The carrots found in this recipe are packed with vitamin A, the power vitamin for pregnancy that is important for your baby's embryonic growth. Vitamin A supports the growth of your baby's kidneys, lungs, heart, eyes, and bones. Therefore, this juice is a spectacular addition to your—and your baby's—day.

YIELDS: 1¼ CUPS

3 carrots, peeled
1 cucumber, peeled
2 beets, greens removed
1 stalk celery, leaves intact

Juice ingredients in order listed. Stir.

	Calories	Fat	Protein	Sodium	Fiber	Carbohydrates
PER 1¼ CUP SERVING	244	0.48g	7.8g	292mg	16g	69g

Super Berry

Good for strengthening your immune system

You've heard it before: Blueberries are powerhouses of antioxidants and vitamin C, so they can build and protect your immune system. They also can help your urinary tract, in a way similar to cranberries.

1 pint blueberries, washed
2 cups red grapes, washed

Juice blueberries and grapes. Stir.

	Calories	Fat	Protein	Sodium	Fiber	Carbohydrates
PER 1 CUP SERVING	288	1.6g	4.1g	6.6mg	7.5g	74g

SUPER BLUEBERRIES

Blueberries are being touted as one of the new superfoods. Their color contains anthocyanin, a phytonutrient that helps reduce cancer risk by preventing cell damage. They are packed with antioxidants and phytoflavinoids and are also high in potassium and vitamin C. Blueberries are not only good for lowering your risk of heart disease and cancer; they are anti-inflammatory and can help eliminate any inflammation that naturally occurs in pregnancy.

200   PART 2: The Recipes

Carrots in the Veggie Patch

Good for your baby's bones and development

The spinach, turnip greens, and celery found in this recipe make this juice a great calcium source to help out with the development of your growing baby. In fact, turnips are rich in calcium and iron, and have two times the vitamin C of orange juice. These nutrients will support the growth of your baby's bones, protect your baby's cells from damage, and protect his immune system.

YIELDS: 1 CUP

2 carrots, peeled
1 cup spinach
1 turnip, including turnip greens
1 stalk celery
2 sprigs parsley

Juice carrots, spinach, turnip, and celery. Stir and garnish with parsley sprigs.

	Calories	Fat	Protein	Sodium	Fiber	Carbohydrates
PER 1 CUP SERVING	160	0.3g	5.2g	266mg	11g	40g

HEALTHY CARROTS

Carrots have been beloved for more than 2,000 years for their good health properties and high vitamin A content. They appear in many juice recipes because they are so healthy. They juice very well, and complement the flavors of other fruits and vegetables quite nicely.

Apple Blackberry

Good for your baby's bones and development

Blackberries contain folate, which helps prevent several birth defects and decreases the rate of miscarriage. However, pesticides and fertilizers used on blackberries can increase the risk of birth defects, so be sure to purchase organic and wash your fruit before juicing.

YIELDS: ¾ CUP

2 Gala red apples, cored
2 pints blackberries
1 lemon, peeled

Juice apples, blackberries, and lemon. Stir.

	Calories	Fat	Protein	Sodium	Fiber	Carbohydrates
PER ¾ CUP SERVING	353	3.4g	8.6g	8.6mg	36g	87g

A Pear of Kiwifruit

Good for fighting infections during pregnancy

One small kiwifruit contains as much vitamin C as a whole orange, which makes it a tasty way to fight infections during pregnancy. Kiwifruits are also full of the flavonoids, beta-carotene, and potassium that keep you and your baby healthy.

YIELDS: ¾ CUP

2 pears
2 kiwi fruit, peeled
½ lemon, peeled

Juice pears, kiwifruit, and lemon. Stir.

	Calories	Fat	Protein	Sodium	Fiber	Carbohydrates
PER ¾ CUP SERVING	222	2.5g	3.3g	6mg	15g	57g

Peach Grape Delight

Peaches have several flavonoids that act as protective scavengers of harmful free radicals that may be looking to cause damage to cells throughout your body. They are also rich in potassium, an important component of cell and body fluids that regulate your blood pressure and can help keep you from developing preeclampsia, high blood pressure in a pregnant woman that can lead to risk of complications for the mother or baby. Therefore, it is important to do everything you can to manage blood pressure throughout your pregnancy.

YIELDS: 1½ CUPS

2 peaches

1 cup red grapes

¼ lemon

Juice peaches, grapes, and lemon. Stir.

	Calories	Fat	Protein	Sodium	Fiber	Carbohydrates
PER 1½ CUP SERVING	188	1.1g	3.9g	2.1mg	7.5g	47g

Fresh from the Garden

Good for your baby's bones and development

The celery and broccoli found in this recipe are full of calcium, which will help your baby's bones develop. The tomato, celery, and broccoli in this refreshing drink will also provide other essential pregnancy nutrients, such as vitamin C and folic acid, that are needed for your baby's growth and development.

1 large tomato

2 stalks celery

1 cup broccoli

2 cloves garlic

Juice tomato, celery, broccoli, and garlic. Stir.

	Calories	Fat	Protein	Sodium	Fiber	Carbohydrates
PER 1¼ CUP SERVING	99	0.0g	6.3g	126mg	6.6g	19g

Tangy Cucumber

Good for morning sickness

The ginger in this juice will alleviate your morning sickness, which makes this spicy drink a blessing in disguise! But it doesn't stop there. The folate-packed cucumbers found in this juice also work to reduce the risk of birth defects. A win-win!

YIELDS: ½ CUP

2 cucumbers

1 lemon, peeled

¼" slice ginger

Pinch kosher salt

Juice cucumbers, lemon, and ginger. Stir in a pinch of salt.

	Calories	Fat	Protein	Sodium	Fiber	Carbohydrates
PER ½ CUP SERVING	119	1.1g	7.3g	156mg	12g	36g

Orange Broccoli

Helps boost energy levels

This juice is a good source of manganese for glucose metabolism, which will ensure that the nutrients from your food are getting to your cells for energy. In addition, broccoli contains a substance called sulforaphane, which produces enzymes that protect blood vessels and helps to reduce cell damage. In order for your baby to grow to the best of her ability, you will need to support an environment that has as little cell damage as possible, so drink up to promote cell growth!

YIELDS: ¾ CUP

2 oranges, peeled
1 cup broccoli, washed

Juice oranges and broccoli. Stir well.

	Calories	Fat	Protein	Sodium	Fiber	Carbohydrates
PER ¾ CUP SERVING	160	0.93g	5.5g	30mg	8.4g	40g

String Bean Juice

Helps boost energy levels

String beans are an excellent source of vitamin B$_6$, which helps increase energy levels by converting your food into energy. If you're slogging through your third trimester, this juice may help boost your energy levels. How? It's full of great sources of fiber like string beans and Brussels sprouts, which help regulate your blood sugars, energy levels, and hunger.

YIELDS: ¾ CUP

1 cup string beans

6 Brussels sprouts

1 lemon, peeled

Juice beans, Brussels sprouts, and lemon. Stir.

	Calories	Fat	Protein	Sodium	Fiber	Carbohydrates
PER ¾ CUP SERVING	118	1.4g	7g	44mg	10g	29g

Carrot Cauliflower

This tasty juice provides you with iron and vitamins A and C. Iron is a crucial mineral during pregnancy as you need more of it to make more hemoglobin as the blood in your body increases to provide protection for your baby. During the second and third trimesters, you'll also need more iron for your growing baby and placenta. Vitamins A and C will also support your baby's growth and bones.

YIELDS: 1½ CUPS

1 cup cauliflower
3 carrots, peeled
1 stalk celery

Juice cauliflower, carrots, and celery. Stir.

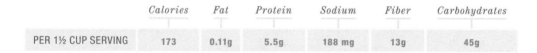

	Calories	Fat	Protein	Sodium	Fiber	Carbohydrates
PER 1½ CUP SERVING	173	0.11g	5.5g	188 mg	13g	45g

CAULIFLOWER OR CABBAGE?

Mark Twain said, "Cauliflower is nothing but cabbage with a college education." It is part of the cabbage family and comes from the Latin words *caulis* for stalk and *floris* for flower. Cauliflower comes in white, orange, green, and purple varieties. The green leaves at the base of the cauliflower are edible. They have a stronger flavor than the curd.

Broccoli Carrot

Good for your baby's bones and development

This juice supplies calcium and vitamins A and C for a perfect combination of nutrients for your baby's growth. These vitamins support bone growth and tissue repair and vitamin C is needed for your body to make collagen that will help develop your baby's bones, skin, and tendons.

YIELDS: 1 CUP

3 carrots, peeled

6 spears broccoli

1 clove garlic

¼ lemon, peeled

Juice carrots, broccoli, and garlic. Juice lemon.

	Calories	Fat	Protein	Sodium	Fiber	Carbohydrates
PER 1 CUP SERVING	195	0.92g	9.1g	175mg	14g	45g

Apple Cabbage

Good for your baby's bones and development

Cabbage and apples are a great combination with wonderful health benefits for you and your baby. Cabbage is a good source of folic acid, which protects your baby from neurological birth defects, and apples will support your digestive system. Not to mention the fact that this juice is pretty delicious to boot!

YIELDS: 1¼ CUPS

¼ head red cabbage
1 cup Napa cabbage
2 Granny Smith apples, cored

Juice ingredients in order listed. Stir.

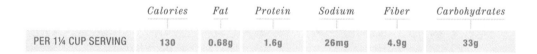

	Calories	Fat	Protein	Sodium	Fiber	Carbohydrates
PER 1¼ CUP SERVING	130	0.68g	1.6g	26mg	4.9g	33g

CABBAGE

A head of cabbage should feel heavy and should have tightly packed leaves. Store in the refrigerator tightly wrapped in plastic for one week. Napa cabbage has a crinkly leaf. It does not have the strong flavor of regular cabbage and is very crisp. Its flavor is mild.

Cucumber Melon Pear

Good for your baby's bones and development

One cup of honeydew melon provides 32mcg of folic acid, which decreases the risk of birth defects in your unborn baby. There are 2 cups of melon used in this recipe, which will give you about 62mcg of folic acid. You need about 400mcg per day, so get juicing!

1 cucumber, washed and peeled
½ melon (honeydew or cantaloupe), rind removed
1 pear

Juice cucumber, melon, and pear. Stir.

	Calories	Fat	Protein	Sodium	Fiber	Carbohydrates
PER 1 CUP SERVING	203	0.77g	4.1g	68mg	8.7g	58g

Green Apple Broccoli

Good for your baby's bones and development

Broccoli is rich in calcium and vitamins A and C, which will help your baby's bones grow strong. It is also high in bioflavonoids and iron. Bioflavonoids and iron can enhance your immune system and ensure that the oxygen from food is delivered to other parts of your body that need it, like your fetus.

6 spears broccoli

3 Granny Smith apples

⅛ cup Italian parsley

1. Juice broccoli, then apples.
2. Add Italian parsley to juicer.
3. Stir and garnish with extra sprig of Italian parsley.

	Calories	Fat	Protein	Sodium	Fiber	Carbohydrates
PER 1½ CUP SERVING	253	1.4g	5.1g	60mg	13g	41g

BROCCOLI

Broccoli is a relative of the cabbage family. It is available year round but peaks from October through April. Keep it refrigerated for up to four days.

Peach Pineapple

Good for your baby's bones and development

Peaches are full of folic acid, and vitamins A and C. Folic acid will support your baby's DNA and prevent neurological birth defects and vitamins A and C will build strong bones for your baby. All that *and* it tastes like peaches and pineapples? Enjoy!

YIELDS: 1½ CUPS

1 cup pineapple

1 peach, washed

Juice pineapple and peach. Stir.

	Calories	Fat	Protein	Sodium	Fiber	Carbohydrates
PER 1½ CUP SERVING	131	0.52g	3.1g	1.6mg	3.1g	35g

PEACHES

Peaches are available from May to October in the United States. The color of the peach's skin ranges from light pinkish white to a yellow gold. Peaches bruise very easily, so try to select ones that do not have soft spots.

Apple Grapefruit

Grapefruit is a good source of vitamin C, also known as ascorbic acid, which is essential for tissue repair, bone growth, fighting infection, and protecting cells from damage to promote the growth of a healthy baby. However, grapefruit has been shown to slightly increase estrogen levels, so talk to your doctor before consuming this juice during pregnancy.

YIELDS: 1 CUP

2 red apples
½ pink grapefruit, rind removed

Juice apples and grapefruit. Stir.

	Calories	Fat	Protein	Sodium	Fiber	Carbohydrates
PER 1 CUP SERVING	167	1.2g	0.69g	2.5mg	6.2g	33g

GRAPEFRUIT

Grapefruit is available year round. Choose grapefruit with thin skin, which has a fine texture. Do not store grapefruit at room temperature for more than one day. However, you may keep them for up to two weeks in your refrigerator. They are best stored in a plastic bag in the vegetable drawer.

Cucumber Pepper

Bell (sweet) peppers are an excellent source of vitamins A and C, that promote bone growth and infection resistance. You have to provide your baby with these vitamins in order to support the growth of his heart, lungs, kidneys, eyes, and bones. In addition, this recipe uses cucumber, which is beneficial in more ways than one. In fact, recent studies have also found that cucumbers might lower the risk for infants to get type 1 diabetes if cucumbers are consumed while the mother was pregnant.

YIELDS: 1 CUP

1 cucumber, washed and peeled
1 stalk celery, washed
½ green bell pepper, washed

Juice cucumbers, celery, and pepper. Stir.

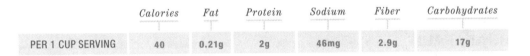

	Calories	Fat	Protein	Sodium	Fiber	Carbohydrates
PER 1 CUP SERVING	40	0.21g	2g	46mg	2.9g	17g

Asparagus Squash Medley

Helps boost energy levels

Squash is high in niacin and vitamins A and C, which will support your baby's bones and immune system, and asparagus restores normal blood sugar levels and energy levels. The high water content in both of these veggies will promote hydration important for the optimal health of you and your baby, making them perfect for juicing during your pregnancy.

YIELDS: 1 CUP

4 spears asparagus
1 cup yellow crookneck squash

Juice asparagus and squash. Stir.

	Calories	Fat	Protein	Sodium	Fiber	Carbohydrates
PER 1 CUP SERVING	51	0g	6.1g	127mg	5.3g	9g

Super Green Juice

Good for your baby's bones and development

This juice is an excellent source of vitamin A and folate, which comes from many sources including the romaine, cucumber, and carrot! One serving and you'll be very close to reaching your daily needs.

YIELDS: 1½ CUPS

1 red apple

4 leaves romaine lettuce, washed

1 cucumber, washed and peeled

1 stalk celery, leaves intact, washed

1 carrot, washed and peeled

1 clove garlic

Juice ingredients in the order listed in the recipe. Stir.

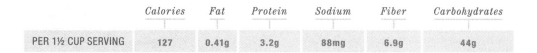

	Calories	Fat	Protein	Sodium	Fiber	Carbohydrates
PER 1½ CUP SERVING	127	0.41g	3.2g	88mg	6.9g	44g

ROMAINE LETTUCE

Romaine originated on the Aegean Island of Kos. Sometimes you will see romaine lettuce referred to as Kos lettuce. It has dark green leaves on the outside and pale green in the center and is commonly used in Caesar salad.

Kiwifruit Apple

Good for your digestive system

This juice contains actinidin, a digestive enzyme found in kiwifruit that will support your digestion throughout your pregnancy by breaking food down in your stomach. Kiwifruit is also a good source of vitamin C that supports tissue repair and bone growth and fights infections during pregnancy.

YIELDS: 1 CUP

2 red apples, washed, cored, and sliced

3 kiwifruit

Juice apples and kiwifruit. Stir.

	Calories	*Fat*	*Protein*	*Sodium*	*Fiber*	*Carbohydrates*
PER 1 CUP SERVING	231	3g	2.7g	9.4mg	11g	64g

KIWI

Another name for kiwifruit is Chinese gooseberry.

Orange Carrot

Good for your baby's bones and development

Beyond helping your body fight infection, vitamin C is essential for tissue repair, bone growth and repair, and healthy skin. The vitamin C in this recipe comes from carrots and oranges and is beneficial for both you and your baby-to-be.

YIELDS: 1 CUP

3 carrots, washed and peeled

1 orange, washed and cut into wedges

Juice carrots and orange. Stir.

	Calories	Fat	Protein	Sodium	Fiber	Carbohydrates
PER 1 CUP SERVING	206	0.31g	4.4g	117mg	12g	55g

CAROTENE

Carrots contain more beta-carotene than any other vegetable. Beta-carotene is converted, only when needed, into vitamin A, which is used directly by the body. Vitamin A is one of the crucial vitamins during pregnancy for developing the heart, lungs, kidneys, eyes, and bones of your baby.

Berry Melon

Good for your baby's bones and development

Strawberries are an excellent source of folic acid, or folate, which helps the body make healthy new cells. It also reduces the chance of some birth defects, such as spina bifida. Not to mention, strawberries are fresh, delicious, and a perfect accompaniment to the cantaloupe in this recipe.

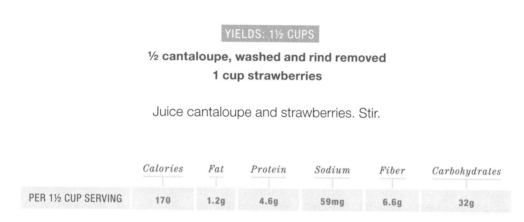

YIELDS: 1½ CUPS

½ cantaloupe, washed and rind removed

1 cup strawberries

Juice cantaloupe and strawberries. Stir.

	Calories	Fat	Protein	Sodium	Fiber	Carbohydrates
PER 1½ CUP SERVING	170	1.2g	4.6g	59mg	6.6g	32g

WHAT IS THE WATER CONTENT OF YOUR FRUIT JUICE?

The water in your fruit isn't your ordinary water. It is full of vitamins, minerals, enzymes, and electrolytes. Fruit juices will refresh and restore your body, helping it reach its optimal level of health to develop a healthy baby.

Cucumber Lemonade

Helps boost energy levels

This hydrating juice will leave you feeling refreshed and energized. Why? Well, the cucumber's high water content makes it excellent for replacing fluids lost through sweating and will help prevent dehydration or exhaustion. Sweating can be more common during pregnancy due to hormonal changes and carrying around a larger body mass, so do whatever you can to stay dry.

YIELDS: 1 CUP

2 cucumbers, washed and peeled

1 lemon, washed, rind removed

Juice cucumbers and lemon. Stir.

	Calories	Fat	Protein	Sodium	Fiber	Carbohydrates
PER 1 CUP SERVING	65	0.2g	2.6g	9.2mg	3.8g	30g

LEMONS

Lemon juice is a natural diuretic that helps eliminate excess fluids that may lead to edema during pregnancy.

Super Melon

The delicious, refreshing fruit used in this recipe are rich in beta-carotene, vitamin C, and potassium. Beta-carotene will convert into vitamin A when needed and will help support the development of your baby's eyes, bones, kidneys, lungs, and heart. The vitamin C will support your and your baby-to-be's immune systems and will protect him from free radical damage, which will enhance her ability to grow into a healthy baby.

YIELDS: 1½ CUPS

1 cup watermelon, rind removed
1 cup cantaloupe, rind removed
1 orange, rind removed

Juice melons and orange. Stir.

	Calories	Fat	Protein	Sodium	Fiber	Carbohydrates
PER 1½ CUP SERVING	164	0.83g	4.5g	27mg	4.4g	43g

CANTALOUPE OR MUSK MELON?

Cantaloupe was named for a castle in Italy. Real cantaloupe is from Europe and is not exported. The American cantaloupes are really known as musk melons. Cantaloupes should have a netting appearance on a beige-colored skin when they are ripe.

Blueberry Banana

Good for fighting infections during pregnancy

Berries are blood purifiers and can help you out during your pregnancy by improving your body's ability to deliver oxygen from your blood to cells that are required for you and your baby's growth and development. Berries also contain antioxidants, which protect your body from bladder infections, high blood pressure, and fatigue, all of which you may experience throughout the various trimesters.

YIELDS: 1½ CUPS

2 cups blueberries, washed

1 banana, peeled

1. Juice blueberries.
2. Blend blueberry juice and banana in juicer.
3. Stir.

	Calories	*Fat*	*Protein*	*Sodium*	*Fiber*	*Carbohydrates*
PER 1½ CUP SERVING	241	1.2g	3.8g	3.7mg	8g	59g

BLUEBERRIES

Low in calories (½ cup has just 40 calories) and high in antioxidants, these sweet yet tart fruits pack a nutritious punch. Blueberries also protect against short-term memory loss, lower cholesterol, and enhance memory. However, most importantly, they are highest in antioxidants to protect you and your baby from free radicals that may damage cells.

Apple Beeter

Good for your baby's bones and development

Apples are a good source of calcium, potassium, folate, and vitamins A and C. Folate is necessary for the production and maintenance of new cells and prevention of birth defects. Today, it is recommended to choose organic apples over industrial apples, because of industrial apples' exposure to an organophosphate pesticide, which is shown to decrease intelligence and increase attention problems in children.

YIELDS: 1 CUP

2 red apples, washed, cored
1 beet, washed, greens removed

Juice apples and beet. Stir.

	Calories	Fat	Protein	Sodium	Fiber	Carbohydrates
PER 1 CUP SERVING	101	0.46g	1.7g	66mg	5g	32g

IS THERE A BITTER TASTE TO YOUR JUICE?

If any of your juices are too bitter for your taste, apples are a perfect sweetener.

Celery Carrot

This juice will help you reach your daily needs for vitamin C, potassium, and folic acid. It can also balance your fluids to avoid any unnecessary fluid retention. If you experience an excess of fluid retention in your body during pregnancy, you are at a higher risk for having high blood pressure, which can lead to preeclampsia.

YIELDS: 1 CUP

3 carrots, peeled
2 stalks celery, leaves intact

Juice carrots and celery. Stir.

	Calories	Fat	Protein	Sodium	Fiber	Carbohydrates
PER 1 CUP SERVING	155	0.23g	4g	198mg	11g	40g

CARROTS

Baby carrots are full of flavor, but because they are not totally mature they are not as flavorful as full-grown carrots. It is important to remove carrot greens before storing them, because keeping them on robs the carrot of moisture and vitamins.

Watermelon Orange

Good for your digestive system

Pregnancy can invite fluids into places that you don't necessarily want swollen. Eating foods that can be used as diuretics is helpful in managing water retention or bloating. Some of these foods are watermelon, garlic, cantaloupe, and dill.

YIELDS: 1¼ CUPS

1 cup watermelon

1 orange, peeled

Juice watermelon and orange. Stir.

	Calories	Fat	Protein	Sodium	Fiber	Carbohydrates
PER 1¼ CUP SERVING	110	0.48g	2.9g	1.5mg	2.8g	28g

MINI MELONS

Watermelons are now available in small individual sizes. They are about the size of a cantaloupe melon. To cut up a melon, you may want to use a melon baller, a small bowl-shaped tool to cut rounds of melon. These can be placed on a skewer and used to decorate your juice.

Broccoli Cabbage Patch

Good for fighting infections during pregnancy

Cabbage is a cruciferous vegetable and contains some vitamin A and a good amount of vitamin C, which will ward off any germ coming your way during pregnancy. The word "cabbage" means "head." Brussels sprouts, broccoli, cauliflower, and kale are all members of the cabbage family.

YIELDS: 1½ CUPS

1 cup broccoli, washed
¼ small head red cabbage, washed
3 leaves romaine lettuce, washed and dried

1. Juice broccoli.
2. Juice cabbage and lettuce.
3. Stir.

	Calories	Fat	Protein	Sodium	Fiber	Carbohydrates
PER 1½ CUP SERVING	48	0.41g	3.3g	43mg	4g	9.6g

Green Juice

Good for pregnancy cravings

There are several cravings during pregnancy that may surprise you, such as a desire for limes, greens, or pepper rings. Sometimes our bodies crave sour foods due to a lack of acetic acid. Green vegetables are high in chlorophyll and help with these types of cravings.

YIELDS: 1½ CUPS

3 stalks celery, leaves
  intact

½ cucumber

1 red apple, washed and
  cored

1 fistful spinach

1 fistful beet greens

1. Wash vegetables.
2. Juice ingredients in the order listed.
3. Stir.

	Calories	Fat	Protein	Sodium	Fiber	Carbohydrates
PER 1½ CUP SERVING	111	0.9g	4.7g	237mg	8.7g	25g

CELERY

Celery is available year round. It is used in many juice recipes because of its sodium. Celery keeps very well in the refrigerator when wrapped in foil and stored in the vegetable drawer.

Carrot Beeter

Good for strengthening your immune system

The beets and carrots in this juice will give you—and your baby-to-be!—a definite immune boost. In addition, carrots have been known to improve the quality of breast milk in mothers and beets provide a good source of magnesium, which can help to reduce cholesterol.

YIELDS: 1¼ CUPS

3 carrots, washed and peeled
1 beet, washed, greens cut off

Juice carrots and then beet. Stir.

	Calories	Fat	Protein	Sodium	Fiber	Carbohydrates
PER 1¼ CUP SERVING	177	0.19g	4.7g	182mg	12g	46g

Piece of Pie

There is now a new meaning to having an apple a day, especially when pregnant. Studies have suggested that by eating an apple every day, you may be able to reduce the risk of your baby developing asthma. This sweet combination can also satisfy your cravings while you enjoy a tasty treat.

YIELDS: 1½ CUPS

3 Granny Smith apples, washed and cored

1 teaspoon cinnamon

1. Juice apples.
2. Add cinnamon and stir.

	Calories	Fat	Protein	Sodium	Fiber	Carbohydrates
PER 1½ CUP SERVING	136	0.63g	0.09g	3.1mg	6.2g	37g

CINNAMON

Cinnamon comes from the inner bark of a tropical evergreen tree and was once used as a love potion in ancient Rome. Today, we tend to associate cinnamon with sweet recipes, but it is quite good in savory stews—or juices and smoothies—as well!

Apple Yammer

Good for strengthening your immune system

This juice offers you a great way to satisfy your sweet tooth while keeping you healthy and supplying your baby with plenty of vitamins A and C, which will help protect your immune systems.

YIELDS: 1 CUP

1 yam, washed and cut into pieces
1 red apple, washed and cored

Juice yam and apple. Stir.

	Calories	Fat	Protein	Sodium	Fiber	Carbohydrates
PER 1 CUP SERVING	232	0.59g	2.8g	14mg	8.2g	51g

SWEET POTATO OR YAM?

Sweet potatoes are part of the morning glory family. In the United States there are many varieties, but the two main ones are a pale sweet potato and the orange-skinned variety known as yams. The true yam is not related to the sweet potato. Do not refrigerate yams, because they will develop a hard core and their flavor will deteriorate.

Garlic Melon with Sprig of Dill

Good for your baby's nervous system

Garlic is a very good source of vitamin B$_6$ and vitamin C that will help develop your baby's nervous system and are essential for tissue and bone repair and bone growth. Garlic is also an old-fashioned cure for water retention, which may come in handy during your pregnancy.

YIELDS: 1 CUP

¼ **cantaloupe, rind removed**
2 **whole cloves garlic**
Sprigs fresh baby dill

1. Juice cantaloupe and garlic.
2. Stir and garnish glass with dill.

	Calories	Fat	Protein	Sodium	Fiber	Carbohydrates
PER 1 CUP SERVING	86	0.57g	2.8g	32mg	2.1g	24g

GARLIC

Garlic is said to provide and prolong strength in the body, and it's also been used as a cure for toothaches. It is a member of the lily family and a cousin of leeks, chives, shallots, and onions. The white-skinned variety is known as American garlic. The Mexican and Italian garlic have a mauve-colored skin and a mild flavor.

Index

Note: Page numbers in **bold** indicate smoothies, and page numbers in *italics* indicate juices.

Almond milk, **43**, **46**, **62**, **64**, **69**, **71**, **74**, **76**, **78**, **82**, **85**, **87**, **88**
Apples
   about: nutritional benefits, 13
   Apple Banana, *151*
   Apple Banana High, *179*
   Apple Beeter, *225*
   Apple Blackberry, *202*
   Apple Cabbage, *211*
   Apple Celery, *150*
   Apple Celery Smoothie, **132**
   Apple Cucumber with a
      Twist, *194*
   Apple-Ginger Delight, **73**
   Apple Grape, *148*
   Apple Grapefruit, *215*
   Apple Lemonade, *149*
   Apple Pie Smoothie, **34**
   Apple Yammer, *232*
   Apricot Apple, *192*
   A Bitter-Sweet Treat, **65**
   Broccoli Apple Carrot, *197*
   Butternut Delight, *187*
   Cabbage Juice, *139*
   Carrot Apple Broccoli, *160*
   Cranberry Apple, *140*
   Folate-Filled Fruit Smoothie,
      119
   Garlic Delight, *198*
   Ginger Carrot Apple, *190*
   Great Granny Smith, **92**
   Green Apple Broccoli, *213*
   The Green Go-Getter, **42**
   Immune Booster, *142*

Kale Apple, *134*
Kale Apple Spinach, *153*
Kiwifruit Apple, *219*
Pear Apple, *193*
Piece of Pie, *231*
Pleasurable Pregnancy
   Smoothie, **114**
The Pregnancy Helper, **64**
Spinach Apple, *186*
Stomach Soother, **57**
Strawberry Patch, *168*
Sunshine in a Glass, *155*
Super Green Juice, *218*
Wake Up Watercress
   Smoothie, **177**
Apricot Apple, *192*
Arugula, **60**, **94**, **99**, **103**, **120**
Asparagus, **95**, **109**, *217*

Bananas
   about: avoiding browning
      of, 135; as thickening
      agent, 32
   Apple Banana, *151*
   Apple Banana High, *179*
   Banana Nut Blend, **85**
   Berry and Banana Smoothie,
      126
   Berry Bananas, **87**
   Berry Happy Mama, **61**
   Blueberry Banana, *224*
   Carrot Banana, *135*
   Chocolatey Dream, **78**
   Coconut Cream Smoothie, **82**

Creamy, Nutty, Sweet
   Smoothie, **59**
Go Bananas, **32**
Great Granny Smith, **92**
The Pregnancy Helper, **64**
Rise and Shine, *191*
Strawberry Papaya, *145*
Basil, **53**, **54**, **66**
Beets and beet greens
   about: beet colors, **100**;
      greens, 74; nutritional
      benefits, 15, 74
   Apple Beeter, *225*
   Beet Booster, **70**
   Broccoli and Kale, *185*
   Carrot Beeter, *230*
   Carrot, Cucumber, and
      Beet, *199*
   Ginger Carrot Beet, *154*
   Green Juice, *229*
   Savoy Smoothie, **68**
   Sweet and Savory Beet, **100**
   A Sweet Beet Smoothie, **44**
   A Sweet Beet Treat, **74**
Berries
   about: bladder health and,
      76; blueberries, 200, 224;
      nutritional benefits, 13, 15,
      40, 200, 224; for sight, 40
   Apple Banana High, *179*
   Apple Blackberry, *202*
   Berry and Banana Smoothie,
      126
   Berry Bananas, **87**

Berry, Berry Delicious, **71**
Berry Cherry, *152*
A Berry Delicious End to the
   Day, **76**
A Berry Great Morning, **35**
Berry Happy Mama, **61**
Berry Melon, *221*
Blackberry Delight, **124**
Blueberry Banana, *224*
Blueberry Supreme, **86**
Cherry and Blueberry, *161*
Circulatory Smoothie, **56**
Cranberry Apple, *140*
Cranberry Orange, *144*
Cran-Energy Smoothie, **117**
Papaya Delight, *157*
Peach Strawberry, *158*
Peachy Berry, **72**
Pleasurable Pregnancy
   Smoothie, **114**
Purple Cow, *169*
Raspberry Delight, **84**
Raspberry Immune System
   Smoothie, **112**
Razzle Dazzle Berry, *180*
Refreshing Raspberry Blend,
   121
Romaine Pineapple
   Smoothie, **125**
Sinful Strawberry Cream, **83**
Strawberry Papaya, *145*
Strawberry Patch, *168*
Strawberry Pineapple Grape,
   170

Strawberry Start, **40**
Sunshine in a Glass, *155*
Super Berry, *200*
Beta-carotene, 17, 220
Beta-Carotene Cantaloupe
  Smoothie, **123**
Birth defects, preventing. *See*
  also Bones and development
  (baby), recipes good for
  folate for, 13, 28, 119, *153*
  juices for, *153, 158, 159,*
    202, 206, 211, 212, 214,
    221, 225
  smoothies for, *43*, **83**, *102*
Blender, choosing, 21
Bones and development (baby),
  recipes good for
  about: overview of, 28
  Apple Beeter, *225*
  Apple Blackberry, *202*
  Apple Cabbage, *211*
  Berry Melon, *221*
  Blazing Broccoli, **96**
  Broccoli Carrot, *210*
  Butternut Delight, *187*
  Cabbage Carrot, **102**
  Carrot Apple Broccoli, *160*
  Carrots in the Veggie Patch,
    201
  Carrot Top of the Morning to
    You, **33**
  Cucumber Melon Pear, *212*
  Fresh from the Garden, *205*
  A Grape Way to Bone Health,
    127
  Kale Carrot Combo, **97**
  Mango Supreme, **89**
  Orange Carrot, *220*
  Peach Pineapple, *214*
  Pleasantly Pear, **45**
  Salad in a Glass, *166*
  Savory Spinach, **115**

Sinful Strawberry Cream, **83**
Splendid Melon, *49*
Strawberry Start, **40**
Super Green Juice, *218*
Veggie Variety, **93**
Book overview, 8–9
Brain food, 38
Broccoli
  about, 213; nutritional
    benefits, 15, 18; storing,
    213
  Blazing Broccoli, **96**
  Broccoli and Kale, *185*
  Broccoli Apple Carrot, *197*
  Broccoli Cabbage Patch, *228*
  Broccoli Carrot, *210*
  Cabbage, Broccoli, and
    Celery, **111**
  Carrot Apple Broccoli, *160*
  Cauliflower Broccoli, *183*
  Fresh from the Garden, *205*
  Green Apple Broccoli, *213*
  Imperative Iron, **109**
  Orange Broccoli, *207*
  Salad in a Glass, *166*
  Savoy and Broccoli, *163*
Brussels sprouts, *208*
B vitamins, 12–14. *See also*
  Folic acid (folate)

Cabbage
  about: cauliflower and, 209;
    vitamin K and, 68
  Apple Cabbage, *211*
  Broccoli Cabbage Patch, *228*
  Cabbage, Broccoli, and
    Celery, **111**
  Cabbage Carrot, **102**
  Cabbage Juice, *139*
  Oh, Sweet Cabbage, **67**
  Savoy and Broccoli, *163*
  Savoy Smoothie, **68**

Tempting Tomato, **50**
Calcium, 14–15
Calorie intake, 12, 116
Cantaloupe. *See* Melons
Carrots
  about, 226; nutritional
    benefits, 17, *201*
  Baby, Be Happy, **118**
  A Bitter-Sweet Treat, **65**
  Broccoli Apple Carrot, *197*
  Broccoli Carrot, *210*
  Cabbage Carrot, **102**
  Cabbage Juice, *139*
  Carrot and Cauliflower, *175*
  Carrot Apple Broccoli, *160*
  Carrot Banana, *135*
  Carrot Beeter, *230*
  Carrot Cauliflower, *209*
  Carrot, Cucumber, and
    Beet, *199*
  Carrot Kale, *164*
  Carrots in the Veggie Patch,
    201
  Carrot Top of the Morning to
    You, **33**
  Celery Carrot, *226*
  Crazy Carrot, **62**
  Folate-Filled Fruit Smoothie,
    119
  Ginger Carrot Apple, *190*
  Ginger Carrot Beet, *154*
  Go to Sleep Smoothie, *174*
  Immune Booster, *142*
  Imperative Iron, **109**
  Italian Carrot, *189*
  Kale Carrot Combo, **97**
  Lettuce Patch, *162*
  Nightcap Smoothie, *173*
  Oh, Sweet Cabbage, **67**
  Orange Carrot, *220*
  Popeye's Rescue, *136*
  Salad in a Glass, *166*

Snap Pea Smoothie, *165*
A Spicy Assortment, **94**
Super Green Juice, *218*
Sweet and Savory Beet, **100**
Turnip Temptation, **107**
Vegetable Seven, *196*
Very Veggie, **52**
Cauliflower, **111**, *175, 183,*
  196, 209
Celery
  about, 229
  Apple Celery, *150*
  Apple Celery Smoothie, **132**
  Apple Cucumber with a
    Twist, *194*
  Cabbage, Broccoli, and
    Celery, **111**
  Carrots in the Veggie Patch,
    201
  Celery Carrot, *226*
  Cherry Cucumber, *156*
  Dilly of a Cucumber, *159*
  Fresh from the Garden, *205*
  Go to Sleep Smoothie, *174*
  The Green Bloody Mary, **101**
  Green Juice, *229*
  Italian Carrot, *189*
  Nightcap Smoothie, *173*
  Savory Celery Celebration,
    105
  Snap Pea Smoothie, *165*
  Spinach Apple, *186*
  Super Celery, **51**
  Super Green Juice, *218*
  Turnip Temptation, **107**
  Vegetable Seven, *196*
  Veggies for Vitamins, **120**
  Veggie Variety, **93**
  Very Veggie, **52**
Cherries
  Berry Cherry, *152*
  Cherry and Blueberry, *161*

Cherry Cucumber, *156*
Cherry Vanilla Treat, **130**
The Slump Bumper, **69**
Watermelon Lime Cherry,
172
Chocolate (cocoa), **78**, **88**
Cinnamon, 231
Citrus
about: citric acid and flavor,
71; grapefruit, *215*;
lemons, 222; nutritional
benefits, 13, 15; vitamin C
and, 18, 37
Apple Cucumber with a
Twist, *194*
Apple Grapefruit, *215*
Apple Lemonade, *149*
Berry, Berry Delicious, **71**
Circulatory Smoothie, **56**
Citrus Cucumber, *188*
Cranberry Orange, *144*
Cucumber Lemonade, *222*
Good Morning Smoothie, **58**
Grapefruit Star, *184*
Luscious Lemon-Lime, **41**
Maternity Medley, **116**
Moodiness Manipulator, **113**
Orange Broccoli, *207*
Orange Carrot, *220*
Orange Lemonade Lift-Off,
178
Orange You Glad You Got Up
for This?, **37**
Pineapple Tangerine, *181*
Raspberry Immune System
Smoothie, **112**
Splendid Citrus, **38**
Sublime Lime, *63*
Super Melon, *223*
Tangy Cucumber, *206*
Ultimate "C" Energizer, *176*
Vitamin C Pack, **128**

Vitamin C Smoothie, **108**
Watermelon Lime Cherry,
172
Watermelon Orange, *227*
White Grape and Lime, *146*
Cloves, power of, 34
Coconut
Coconut Craziness, **39**
Coconut Cream Smoothie, **82**
The Joy of Almonds, **79**
Coconut milk, 34, 37, 39, 65, 79
Cravings, recipes good for
about: craving sweets and,
73; overview of, 27
Apple-Ginger Delight, **73**
Apple Pie Smoothie, **34**
Banana Nut Blend, **85**
A Berry Delicious End to the
Day, **76**
Berry Happy Mama, **61**
Chocolatey Dream, **78**
Coconut Cream Smoothie, **82**
Creamy, Nutty, Sweet
Smoothie, **59**
Go Nuts for Chocolate!, **88**
The Green Bloody Mary, **101**
The Green Go-Getter, **42**
Green Juice, *229*
The Joy of Almonds, **79**
A Sweet Beet Treat, **74**
Cucumbers
about: storing, 93
Apple Cucumber with a
Twist, *194*
Calming Cucumber, **48**
Carrot, Cucumber, and
Beet, *199*
Cherry Cucumber, *156*
Citrus Cucumber, *188*
A Cool Blend for Pregnancy,
129
Cool Cucumber Melon, **75**

Cucumber Lemonade, *222*
Cucumber Melon Pear, *212*
Cucumber Pepper, *216*
Dilly of a Cucumber, *159*
Green Gazpacho, **66**
Green Juice, *229*
Pineapple Cucumber, *182*
Popeye's Rescue, *136*
Super Green Juice, *218*
Tangy Cucumber, *206*
Tropical Cucumber, *147*
Veggies for Vitamins, **120**
Veggie Variety, **93**

Digestive system, recipes for.
See also Morning sickness,
recipes good for
about: overview of, 26–27
Apple Cucumber with a
Twist, *194*
Apricot Apple, *192*
Citrus Cucumber, *188*
Italian Carrot, *189*
Kiwifruit Apple, *219*
Pear Apple, *193*
Pear Pineapple, *195*
Pear Splendor, *43*
Pineapple Greets Papaya,
138
Pumpkin Spice, **80**
Rise and Shine, *191*
Watermelon Orange, *227*
Dill, *159, 233*

Endive, **49**
Energy-boosting recipes
about: overview of, 27
Apple Celery Smoothie, **132**
Asparagus Squash Medley,
217
Berry Bananas, **87**
A Berry Great Morning, **35**

Cauliflower Broccoli, *183*
A Cool Blend for Pregnancy,
129
Cool Cucumber Melon, **75**
Cran-Energy Smoothie, **117**
Crazy Carrot, *62*
Cucumber Lemonade, *222*
Go Bananas, **32**
Great Garlic, **104**
Green Gazpacho, **66**
Imperative Iron, **109**
Lettuce Patch, *162*
Mango Tango, **36**
Orange Broccoli, *207*
Orange Lemonade Lift-Off,
178
Pineapple Tangerine, *181*
Powerful Pepper Trio, **103**
Refreshing Raspberry Blend,
121
Savoy Smoothie, **68**
The Slump Bumper, **69**
Splendid Citrus, **38**
String Bean Juice, *208*
A Sweet Beet Smoothie, **44**
Ultimate "C" Energizer, *176*
Wake Up Watercress
Smoothie, *177*
Watermelon Straight Up, *141*
Zippy Zucchini, **99**

Fennel, **98**
Folic acid (folate), 12–14, 26,
119

Garlic
about, 233
Fresh from the Garden, *205*
Garlic Delight, *198*
Garlic Melon with Sprig of
Dill, *233*
Go, Go, Garlic!, *53*

Great Garlic, **104**

Vegetable Seven, *196*

Ginger

about: power of, 46

Apple-Ginger Delight, **73**

Ginger and Spice Make
Everything Nice, **46**

Ginger Carrot Apple, *190*

Ginger Carrot Beet, *154*

Ginger Melon Stress
Meltaway, **110**

The Pregnancy Helper, **64**

Stomach Soother, **57**

Tangy Cucumber, *206*

Grapes, **127**, *146*, *148*, *170*, *200*

Greens. *See* Arugula; Lettuce
and greens; Spinach

Healthy pregnancy diet

calorie intake, 12, 116

macro- and micronutrients
for, 12–19

this book and, 8–9

Immune system, strengthening

about: recipes for, 28

Apple Yammer, *232*

A Bitter-Sweet Treat, **65**

Blackberry Delight, **124**

Blueberry Supreme, **86**

Broccoli and Kale, *185*

Carrot Beeter, *230*

Go, Go, Garlic!, **53**

Immune Booster, *142*

Luscious Lemon-Lime, **41**

Orange You Glad You Got Up
for This?, **37**

Raspberry Immune System
Smoothie, **112**

Savoy and Broccoli, *163*

Strawberry Patch, *168*

Strawberry Pineapple Grape,

170

Sublime Lime, **63**

Super Berry, *200*

Vitamin C Smoothie, **108**

Infection-fighting recipes

about: overview of, 29

Berry, Berry Delicious, **71**

Broccoli Cabbage Patch, *228*

Cabbage, Broccoli, and
Celery, **111**

Circulatory Smoothie, **56**

Cranberry Apple, *140*

Cranberry Orange, *144*

A Daring Pearing, **91**

Fantastic Fennel, **98**

Mango Kiwifruit, *137*

A Pear of Kiwifruit, *203*

Strawberry Papaya, *145*

Ingredients. *See also specific
ingredients*

juicing, 22–23

making smoothies, 20–22

organic, 21–22, 72

selecting and storing, 21–22

Iron, 15–16

Juices, 133–233. *See also
specific ingredients*

for baby's bones and
development. *See* Bones
and development (baby),
recipes good for

for baby's nervous system.
See Nervous system
(baby), recipes good for

for cravings. *See* Cravings,
recipes good for

for energy. *See* Energy-
boosting recipes

for fighting infections. *See*
Infection-fighting recipes

juicing, 22–23

for morning sickness. *See*
Morning sickness, recipes
good for

recipes by page number, 6–7

for skin and hair health.
See Skin and hair health,
recipes good for

sweetening, 225

for your digestive system.
See Digestive system,
recipes for

for your immune system.
See Immune system,
strengthening

Kale

Broccoli and Kale, *185*

Carrot Kale, *164*

juices with, *134*, *153*, *164*,
185

Kale Apple Spinach, *153*

smoothies with, **38**, **97**

Kefir, **41**, **61**, **75**, **83**, **117**, **121**,
131

Kiwifruit, *137*, *203*, *219*

Lemon and lime. *See* Citrus

Lettuce and greens. *See also*
Arugula; Beets and beet
greens; Spinach

about: iron and, 16; romaine
lettuce, 218

Awesome Asparagus, **95**

A Berry Great Morning, **35**

Broccoli Cabbage Patch, *228*

Calming Cucumber, **48**

Carrot Top of the Morning to
You, *33*

Coconut Craziness, **39**

Coconut Cream Smoothie, **82**

Crazy Carrot, **62**

Ginger and Spice Make

Everything Nice, **46**

Go, Go, Garlic!, **53**

Go to Sleep Smoothie, *174*

Lettuce Patch, *162*

Luscious Lemon-Lime, **41**

Mango Madness, **47**

Mango Tango, **36**

Nightcap Smoothie, *173*

One Superb Herb, **54**

Orange You Glad You Got Up
for This?, **37**

Pleasantly Pear, **45**

The Pregnancy Helper, **64**

Pregnant Pomegranate
Smoothie, **122**

Raspberry Delight, **84**

Romaine Pineapple
Smoothie, **125**

Salad in a Glass, *166*

Super Green Juice, *218*

Turnip Temptation, **107**

Wacky Watermelon, **77**

Lycopene, 196

Macro- and micronutrients,
12–19

Magnesium, 126

Mangos

about: nutritional benefits, 17

Mango Kiwifruit, *137*

Mango Madness, **47**

Mango Supreme, **89**

Mango Tango, **36**

Rise and Shine, *191*

Tropical Cucumber, *147*

Melons

about: cantaloupes or
musk melons, 223; mini
watermelons, 227; vitamin
C and, 18

Berry Melon, *221*

Beta-Carotene Cantaloupe

Smoothie, **123**
Cantaloupe Straight Up, *171*
Cool Cucumber Melon, **75**
Cran-Energy Smoothie, **117**
Cucumber Melon Pear, *212*
Fresh Start, **55**
Garlic Melon with Sprig of
   Dill, *233*
Ginger Melon Stress
   Meltaway, **110**
Moodiness Manipulator, **113**
Splendid Melon, **49**
Super Melon, *223*
Vitamin C Smoothie, **108**
Wacky Watermelon, **77**
Watermelon and Watercress
   Smoothie, **131**
Watermelon Lime Cherry,
   172
Watermelon Orange, *227*
Watermelon Straight Up, *141*
Milks, vitamin D and, 17. *See
   also* Almond milk; Coconut
   milk; Rice milk; Soymilk
Moodiness Manipulator, **113**
Morning sickness, recipes
   good for. *See also* Digestive
   system, recipes for
      about: overview of, 26
      Fresh Start, **55**
      Ginger and Spice Make
         Everything Nice, **46**
      Ginger Carrot Apple, *190*
      Good Morning Smoothie, **58**
      Great Granny Smith, **92**
      The Pregnancy Helper, **64**
      Stomach Soother, **57**
      Tangy Cucumber, *206*
      Wacky Watermelon, **77**

Nervous system (baby), recipes
   good for

about: overview of, 26
Beet Booster, **70**
Garlic Melon with Sprig of
   Dill, *233*
Just Peachy, **90**
Kale Apple, **134**
Oh, Sweet Cabbage, **67**
One Superb Herb, **54**
Peas for a Perfect Pregnancy,
   60
Raspberry Delight, **84**
Sweet Potato Pie, **81**
Tempting Tomato, **50**
Turnip Temptation, **107**
Very Veggie, **52**
Nutrients (macro and micro),
   12–19, 113. *See also specific
   nutrients*
Nuts and seeds
   about: vitamin D and, 17;
      walnuts and antioxidants,
      85
   Banana Nut Blend, **85**
   Creamy, Nutty, Sweet
      Smoothie, **59**
   Go Nuts for Chocolate!, **88**
   The Joy of Almonds, **79**

Onions, **52**, **66**, **95**, **120**, *166*,
   196
Orange. *See* Citrus
Organic ingredients, 21–22, 72

Pampering yourself, **114**
Papaya, *138*, *145*, *157*
Parsley, **52**, *164*, *174*, *189*,
   196–198, *201*, *213*
Peaches
   about, 214; organic alert, 72
   Just Peachy, **90**
   Peach Grape Delight, *204*
   Peach Pineapple, *214*

Peach Strawberry, *158*
Peachy Berry, **72**
Rise and Shine, *191*
Pears
   about: fiber effects, 45;
      nutritional benefits, 13
   A Cool Blend for Pregnancy,
      129
   Cucumber Melon Pear, *212*
   A Daring Pearing, **91**
   A Grape Way to Bone Health,
      127
   Pear Apple, *193*
   A Pear of Kiwifruit, *203*
   Pear Pineapple, *195*
   Pear Splendor, **43**
   Pleasantly Pear, **45**
   The Slump Bumper, **69**
Peas
   about: nutritional benefits, 50
   Baby, Be Happy, **118**
   Peas for a Perfect Pregnancy,
      60
   Snap Pea Smoothie, *165*
   Tempting Tomato, **50**
Peppers, **66**, **96**, **103**, **115**, *216*
Pineapple
   about: selecting, 167
   Berry and Banana Smoothie,
      126
   Circulatory Smoothie, **56**
   Mango Tango, **36**
   Maternity Medley, **116**
   Papaya Delight, *157*
   Peach Pineapple, *214*
   Pear Pineapple, *195*
   Pineapple Cucumber, *182*
   Pineapple Greets Papaya,
      138
   Pineapple Plum Punch, *167*
   Pineapple Tangerine, *181*
   Raspberry Immune System

Smoothie, **112**
Refreshing Raspberry Blend,
   121
Rise and Shine, *191*
Romaine Pineapple
   Smoothie, **125**
Splendid Citrus, **38**
Strawberry Pineapple Grape,
   170
Tropical Cucumber, *147*
Vitamin C Pack, **128**
Vitamin C Smoothie, **108**
Watermelon and Watercress
   Smoothie, **131**
Plums, in Pineapple Plum
   Punch, *167*
Pomegranate smoothie, **122**
Pumpkin Spice, **80**
Purple Cow, *169*

Radicchio, **44**
Radishes, 16, *143*, *166*
Recipes, callouts, 26–29. *See
   also specific callouts*
Rice milk, **59**, **84**, **86**

Sinus Cleanser, *143*
Skin and hair health, recipes
   good for
      about: overview of, 28
      Apple Banana, *151*
      Apple Celery, *150*
      Mango Madness, **47**
      Peachy Berry, **72**
      Savory Celery Celebration,
         105
      Tropical Cucumber, *147*
Sleep aids, *156*, *173*, *174*
Smoothies, 31–132. *See also
   specific ingredients*
   for baby's bones and
      development. *See* Bones

and development (baby), recipes good for
for baby's nervous system. *See* Nervous system (baby), recipes good for
for cravings. *See* Cravings, recipes good for
for energy. *See* Energy-boosting recipes
for fighting infections. *See* Infection-fighting recipes
making, 20–22
for morning sickness. *See* Morning sickness, recipes good for
recipes by page number, 4–6
for skin and hair health. *See* Skin and hair health, recipes good for
thickening, 32
for your digestive system. *See* Digestive system, recipes for
for your immune system. *See* Immune system, strengthening
Sodium (salt), 18–19
Soymilk, **35**, **40**, **68**, **80**, **81**
Spinach
about: nutritional benefits, 16, 17
Apple Pie Smoothie, **34**
Baby, Be Happy, **118**
Blazing Broccoli, **96**
Carrots in the Veggie Patch, *201*
Cherry Vanilla Treat, **130**
Cran-Energy Smoothie, **117**
A Daring Pearing, **91**
Folate-Filled Fruit Smoothie, **119**
Go Bananas, **32**

Great Garlic, **104**
The Green Go-Getter, **42**
Green Juice, *229*
Imperative Iron, **109**
Kale Apple Spinach, *153*
Lettuce Patch, *162*
Pear Splendor, *43*
Popeye's Rescue, *136*
Savory Spinach, 115
Savory Squash Surprise, **105**
Sinful Strawberry Cream, **83**
The Slump Bumper, **69**
Spinach Apple, *186*
Sublime Lime, **63**
Super Celery, **51**
Veggie Variety, **93**
Very Veggie, **52**
Vitamin C Pack, **128**
Wake Up Watercress Smoothie, *177*
Squash. *See also* Zucchini
about: beta-carotene and, 17
Asparagus Squash Medley, *217*
Butternut Delight, *187*
Pumpkin Spice, **80**
Savory Squash Surprise, **106**
Storing ingredients and smoothies, 21–22
String Bean Juice, *208*
Sweet potatoes and yams, 81, *232*
Swiss chard, iron and, 16

Tomatoes
Fresh from the Garden, *205*
Garlic Delight, *198*
Go, Go, Garlic!, **53**
The Green Bloody Mary, **101**
Green Gazpacho, **66**
Sinus Cleanser, *143*
Tempting Tomato, **50**

Vegetable Seven, *196*
Veggies for Vitamins, **120**
Veggie Variety, **93**
Turnips, **107**, *142*, *201*

Vanilla, in Cherry Vanilla Treat, **130**
Vitamin A, 17
Vitamin B (B vitamins), 12–14. *See also* Folic acid (folate)
Vitamin C, 18, 37. *See also* Citrus
Vitamin D, 17
Vitamin K, 68

Water
content, of fruit juice, 221
intake, 131
Watercress
about: nutritional benefits, 65
Beta-Carotene Cantaloupe Smoothie, **123**
A Bitter-Sweet Treat, **65**
Blackberry Delight, **124**
Chocolatey Dream, **78**
Circulatory Smoothie, **56**
A Cool Blend for Pregnancy, **129**
Creamy, Nutty, Sweet Smoothie, **59**
Fresh Start, **55**
Ginger Melon Stress Meltaway, **110**
Go Nuts for Chocolate!, **88**
Good Morning Smoothie, **58**
A Grape Way to Bone Health, **127**
The Green Bloody Mary, **101**
Green Gazpacho, **66**
Immune Booster, *142*
Maternity Medley, **116**
Moodiness Manipulator, **113**

Pleasurable Pregnancy Smoothie, **114**
Refreshing Raspberry Blend, **121**
Savory Celery Celebration, **105**
Stomach Soother, **57**
Vitamin C Smoothie, **108**
Wake Up Watercress Smoothie, *177*
Watermelon and Watercress Smoothie, **131**
Watermelon. *See* Melons

Yams and sweet potatoes, 81, *232*
Yogurt
blending juices with, 192
nutritional benefits, 44
smoothies with, **44**, **73**, **80**, **82**, **84**, **87**, **124–126**, **129**

Zinc, 18
Zucchini, **94**, **99**

About the Author

Nicole Cormier, RD, LDN, is a registered dietitian, local food enthusiast, and owner of the nutrition counseling company, Delicious Living Nutrition, Inc., and health food store, Farm Fare Market located in Sandwich, Massachusetts. She is also host of *Radio Brunch*, author of *The Everything® Guide to Nutrition* and *The Everything® Healthy College Cookbook*, and the coauthor of *The Everything® Juicing Book* and *201 Healthy Smoothies & Juices for Kids*. Nicole lives in Buzzard's Bay, Massachusetts with her partner Jim Lough, an organic farmer.